THE READING BRAIN
The Biological
Basis of Dyslexia

Edited by Drake D. Duane, M.D.
and David B. Gray, Ph.D.

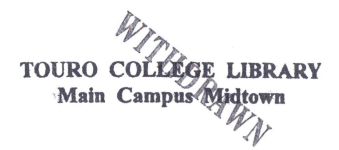

YORK
PRESS

Parkton, Maryland

This book was manufactured in the United States of America. Typography
by Brushwood Graphics, Inc., Baltimore, Maryland. Printing and binding by
McNaughton & Gunn, Inc., Ann Arbor, Michigan. Cover design by Joseph
Dieter, Jr.

Library of Congress Catalog Card Number 91-65273
ISBN 0-912752-25-4

Contents

Participants / iv

Preface / v
    Drake D. Duane and David B. Gray

Introduction / vi
    David B. Gray

Chapter 1
Neurobehavioral Definition of Dyslexia / 1
    Frank Wood, Rebecca Felton, Lynn Flowers, and Cecile Naylor

Chapter 2
Neurolinguistic and Biologic Mechanisms in Dyslexia / 27
    Bennett Shaywitz, Sally Shaywitz, Isabelle Liberman, Jack Fletcher,
    Donald Shankweiler, James Duncan, Leonard Katz, Alvin Liberman,
    David Francis, Lois Dreyer, Stephen Crain, Susan Brady, Anne Fowler,
    Leon Kier, Nancy Rosenfield, John Gore, and Robert Makuch

Chapter 3
Colorado Reading Project
    An Update / 53
    J. C. DeFries, R. K. Olson, B. F. Pennington, and S. D. Smith

Chapter 4
Dyslexia Subtypes
    Genetics, Behavior, and Brain Imaging / 89
    Herbert Lubs, Ranjan Duara, Bonnie Levin, Bonnie Jallad,
    Marie-Louise Lubs, Mark Rabin, Alex Kushch, and Karen Gross-Glenn

Chapter 5
Anatomy of Dyslexia
    Argument Against Phrenology / 119
    Albert Galaburda

Chapter 6
Magnetic Resonance Imaging
    Its Role in the Developmental Disorders / 133
    Pauline Filipek and David Kennedy

Discussion / 161

Summary / 179
    Drake D. Duane

Index / 187

Participants

John C. DeFries, Ph.D.
Institute for Behavioral Genetics
University of Colorado
Campus Box 447
Boulder, CO 80309

Drake D. Duane, M.D.
Director, Institute for
Developmental and Behavioral
Neurology
North Medical Plaza
10250 North 92nd Street, Suite 117
Scottsdale, AZ 85258

Pauline A. Filipek, M.D.
Center for Morphometric Analysis
Massachusetts General Hospital
MGH 13th Street, 6th Floor
Charlestown, MA 02129

Albert M. Galaburda, M.D.
Beth Israel Hospital
Neurological Unit
330 Brookline Avenue
Boston, MA 02215

David B. Gray, Ph.D.
NICHD
Executive Plaza North, Room 631
6130 Executive Boulevard
Bethesda, MD 20892

Herbert Lubs, M.D.
University of Miami School of
Medicine
Department of Pediatrics
Division of Genetics
MCCD P.O. Box 016820
Miami, FL 33101

Bennett A. Shaywitz, M.D.
Professor of Pediatrics
Child Study Center
Yale University School of Medicine
333 Cedar Street
New Haven, CT 06510

Frank Wood, Ph.D.
Professor of Neurology and
Neuropsychology
Section of Neuropsychology
Bowman Gray School of Medicine
300 S. Hawthorne Road
Winston-Salem, NC 27103

Preface

      This volume is a compendium of papers delivered in Dallas, Texas on November 29, 1989 at the annual meeting of The Orton Dyslexia Society. This preconference symposium represents the four NICHD funded Dyslexia Program Projects (Dr. Wood–Bowman-Gray School of Medicine; Dr. DeFries–University of Colorado; Dr. Lubs–University of Miami School of Medicine; Dr. Shaywitz–Yale University School of Medicine) and two NIH funded related projects (Dr. Galaburda–Beth Israel Hospital and Dr. Filipek–Massachusetts General Hospital, both of Harvard Medical School).

This symposium was made possible by a grant guarantee provided by the Curtis Blake Foundation of Springfield, Massachusetts. The support of the Foundation, The Orton Dyslexia Society, and the presenters is gratefully acknowledged.

DDD
Scottsdale, AZ
DBG
Bethesda, MD
September, 1990

Introduction

David B. Gray

The National Institute of Child Health and Human Development (NICHD), a part of the National Institutes of Health (NIH), has funded research in the fields of communication, language, speech, listening, reading, and cognition since the Institute's inception in 1963. The early research had a focus on basic learning, cognitive and perceptual processes. As the attention of educators, clinicians, and legislators turned toward providing individualized educational and therapeutic regimes for all disabled children, the research funded by the NICHD broadened its scope to include studies of children who were classified as dyslexic, attention deficit disordered, hyperactive, and developmental language disordered. Figure 1 provides an illustration of the dramatic growth in NICHD funding of reading related research during the period of 1975 to 1990. Support for research projects directly or indirectly related to specific language disability has grown from 1.75 million dollars in 1975 to 10.42 million dollars in 1990, a cumulative total of 76 million dollars. The specific learning disabilities category is used by the NICHD to track program growth in dyslexia, attention deficit disorders, and hyperactivity and in developmental language disability.

A major impetus for research growth in these areas was the passage of Public Law 94-142—the Education of all Handicapped Children Act in 1978. In 1978 fewer than 5% of the funds distributed by the Office of Special Education Programs (OSEP—an agency within the U.S. Department of Education) were used to provide improved educational services for children with learning disabilities (LD). Within the past decade the number of children categorized by school system criteria as learning disabled has risen from 1% to 5%. The proportion of funds distributed by OSEP for enhancing education for children with LD has

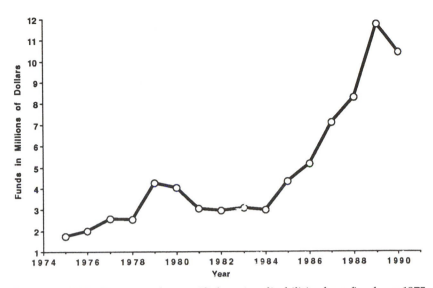

Figure 1.   NICHD support for specific learning disabilities from fiscal year 1975 through 1990.

grown to almost 50% of all OSEP funds or approximately one billion dollars. One basic reason for this change is the continuing lack of agreement on a definition of learning disabilities. The scientific basis for developing a classification system for learning disabilities has not progressed to the point that research scientists can be certain that the samples they study are comparable. As a result of these definitional problems, treatment varies widely from school district to school district. Scientific studies of heterogeneous school referred samples or uniquely homogeneous clinical samples often produce conflicting findings.

In 1983, after reviewing the level and type of research activity supported by the NICHD for studies on dyslexia and related disorders, a discrepancy between biological and behavioral approaches to the study of dyslexia was apparent. The types of research awards were those provided to individual investigators (individual investigator awards or R01) who were doing cutting edge research within a narrow domain of science that is directly or indirectly related to a single aspect of reading, language, neuroanatomy, genetics, electrophysiology, speech, education, visual or auditory perception, or a variety of other fields of science. An exception to the trend of funding individual investigators was the Colorado Reading Project, a program project on studying biological and environmental influences on the acquisition of reading. The program project research award (P01 figure 2a) is a mechanism of NIH funding that requires three or more studies that address a common theme, in this case reading. The Colorado Reading Project

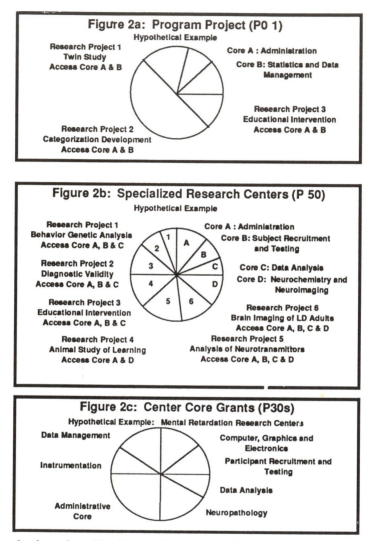

Figure 2 a, b, and c.   Funding mechanisms used by the NICHD for supporting multidisciplinary research.

has utilized the expertise of neuropsychologists, molecular and population geneticists, education specialists, language developmentalists, electrophysiologists, statisticians, mathematicians, and scientists from other disciplines.

The need to address the complexity of etiological factors involved in dyslexia and other learning disabilities through multidisciplinary projects led the NICHD to hold a national conference where leading representatives of a variety of scientific disciplines could discuss the possibilities of working together to develop methods, measures, and sample selection criteria which would allow the results of biological and behavioral studies to be compared. The conference was held in the fall of 1984 at the National Institutes of Health. At the conference, the scientific analysis of dyslexia was described as being further complicated by the differences in the expression of the disability at different ages, the overlap between general and specific cognitive deficits, gender differences, and cultural differences. The proceedings of this conference were published in a book entitled *Biobehavioral Measures of Dyslexia* (Gray and Kavanagh 1985).

As a result of the recommendations made by the participants at this conference, a request for applications (RFA) using the program project funding mechanism that included both biological and behavioral measures of dyselxia to define and subtype dyslexia was published in 1985 (85-HD-10, 1985). Subsequent to this announcement, four program projects were funded. Dr. Frank Wood (see Chapter 1) was funded in 1986 to study the relationships between poor reading and neurological functioning. In 1987, Dr. Bennett Shaywitz (see Chapter 2) was funded to develop a classification scheme for reading, mathematics, and attention deficit disorders of children. Dr. Herbert Lubs (see Chapter 4) received support for a program project in 1987 to investigate the role of genetics in dyslexia. In 1987 Dr. Albert Galaburda (see Chapter 5) was awarded a program project for the purpose of developing animal models of dyslexia and studying neurological characteristics of individuals with dyslexia.

The second major growth in the learning disabilities program occurred when three learning disabilities research centers (LDRCs) were funded in 1989 and 1990. The impetus for these centers originated in the Health Research Extension Act of 1985 (Public Law 99-158) which mandated the establishment of an Interagency Committee on Learning Disabilities (ICLD) for the purpose of reviewing and assessing "Federal research priorities, activities, and findings regarding learning disabilities (including central nervous system dysfunction in children)." The NICHD was designated the lead agency for this congressional initiative. The ICLD held a public forum to solicit input on the nature of the problem and directions for future research. Learning disabled individuals, their families, teachers, administrators, advocacy organizations, practitioners, and scientists made formal presentations to the Committee. In addition, the ICLD collected and analyzed the Federal research support for learning disabilities. In January, 1987, a National Conference on Learning Disabilities was held to discuss the current state of knowledge, identify gaps, and make recommendations for future research. In August of 1987, the Committee's report was submitted to the House of Representatives and the Senate. One of the recommendations contained in "Learning Disabilities: A Report to the U.S. Congress" was to establish multidisciplinary research centers for the study of learning disabilities. On April 8, 1988 the National Institute of Child Health and Human Development (NICHD) announced a request for applications to study learning disabilities from a multidisciplinary perspective (88-HD/NS-1, 1988.)

The objective of this RFA *Learning Disabilities: Multidisciplinary Research Centers* was to develop new knowledge in the fields of etiology, diagnosis, prevention, treatment, and amelioration of learning disabilities. Applications were required to include research on basic biological and behavioral factors relevant to learning disabilities. The major goal of the RFA was to fund intensive multidimensional studies of well defined populations of learning disabled persons. The RFA was designed to encourage applications for research centers that involved the collaboration of a variety of scientists including biologists, neuroscientists, geneticists, epidemiologists, anatomists, psychologists, physicians, educators, linguists, speech and hearing researchers, pharmacologists, demographers, and others. The topics of research to be addressed included, but were not limited to, studies of learning disabled individuals at risk for or exhibiting deficiencies in speech, listening, reading, writing, reasoning, mathematics, and social skills.

In Fiscal Year 1989, with funds specifically provided by Congress, the NICHD awarded two grants for the establishment of two centers in the area of learning disabilities. These centers are located at Yale and The Johns Hopkins Universities. Dr. Bennett Shaywitz of Yale University is the principal investigator of the Yale University Learning Disabilities Research Center (LDRC) *Center for the Study of Learning and Attention Disorders* which addresses the fundamental question of the classification of individuals as learning disabled (figure 3a). If successful, this nosology will provide discriminant and convergent validity for the classification of individuals with learning disabilities, attention deficit disorders, and conduct disorders. This would be a major contribution to the study of learning disabilities by reducing sample heterogeneity and establishing the basis for studying the incidence and prevalence of these disorders.

The second Learning Disabilities Research Center is located at The Johns Hopkins University and is headed by Dr. Martha Bridge Denckla (figure 3b). The goals of this LDRC are to study behavioral aspects of biological etiologies of known genetic anomalies and relate these finding to specific domain deficiencies characteristic of individuals with learning disabilities. Three genetic anomalies (Fragile X, Turner's syndrome, and Tourette's syndrome) will be examined for specific brain behavior deficits that may share fundamental mechanism deficiencies with the more generic forms of learning disabilities. In ad-

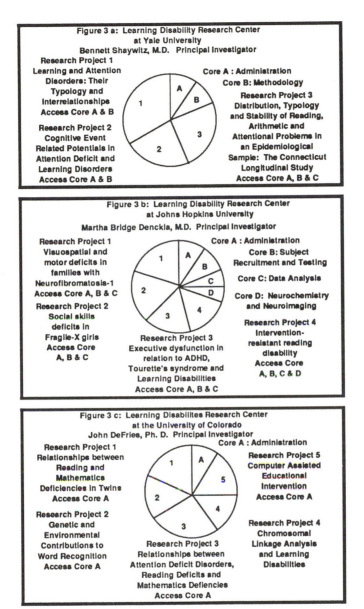

Figure 3 a, b, and c. NICHD funded learning disabilities research centers 1990.

dition, this grantee proposes to examine children whose poor reading is not remediable through normal classroom interventions.

A third LDRC was funded in 1990 in response to a request for applications that had been published on January 19, 1990 (90-HD-02,

1990). The award was made to the University of Colorado. Dr. John DeFries directs this group of scientists who are studying the etiology, course, and remediation of unexpectedly poor performance in reading and mathematics. A large sample of twins (identical and fraternal) and their families are being studied for genetic and environmental contributions to academic achievement in reading and mathematics. Genetic and environmental contributions to specific components of the reading process are being separated through the use of newly developed statistical methods. Chromosomal linkage studies, computer assisted education, and relationships between reading disability and attention deficits are being addressed at this LDRC (see figure 3c).

CURRENT FUNDING OF DYSLEXIA BY NICHD

The NICHD utilizes a variety of funding mechanisms to support research on dyslexia. Support for projects directly related to dyslexia has grown from 2.9 million dollars in 1980 to 7.7 million dollars in 1990 (see figure 4). DeFries, Wood, Lubs, Shaywitz, and Galaburda are currently funded by the program projects mechanism (see figure 2a). The program project mechanism of funding (P01) accounted for 1.3 million dollars of the funding in dyslexia related research in 1980 and has grown to 3.6 million dollars in fiscal year 1990 (figure 5)—a significant increase. Three LDRCs (Yale University, Johns Hopkins, and University of Col-

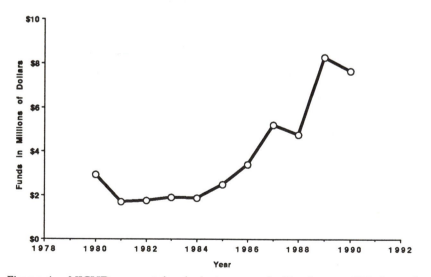

Figure 4. NICHD support for dyslexia research: Fiscal years 1980 through 1990.

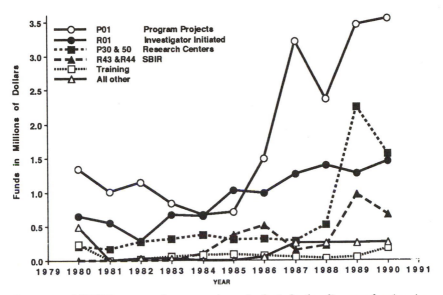

Figure 5. NICHD support for research on dyslexia by funding mechanism in fiscal years 1980–1990.

orado) are funded under the specialized research center mechanism (P50, see figure 2b). As a result of the award of three LDRCs in 1989 and 1990, the center mechanism for funding research has increased while the other mechanisms have used a proportionally lower percent of the funding pie (figure 5). The NICHD funds a small amount of dyslexia related research at the Mental Retardation Research Centers through the core center (P30) mechanism (see figure 2c) for funding dyslexia related researchers. These funds are included in the research centers category in figure 5. The investigator initiated research award mechanism has grown from .7 million dollars of funded research in 1980 to 1.5 million dollars in 1990 (figure 5). Over the past ten years, funding has not increased greatly for investigator initiated research (R01) applications. The Small Business Innovation Research (SBIR) grant award mechanism has been used to develop computer assisted instruction and computer aided assessment of reading. This program began support for dyslexia related research in 1984 with .1 million dollars and has grown to .6 million dollars in 1990 (see figure 5). Very few research training grants have been funded during the past decade (see figure 5). Thus, the program project and center grants can be seen as the primary manner through which the NICHD has provided leadership in bringing learning disabilities research to the attention of the scientific community.

FUTURE DIRECTIONS

The program projects and LDRCs funded by the NICHD are providing funds for multidisciplinary studies of structure function relationships fundamental to the brain's ability to process the written word as reading. At these research sites, new technologies for studying brain morphology and function will be used to address fundamental issues. Some of these include: What theoretical issues might be best addressed by each brain imaging approach and what degree of interface with the results of other procedures is reasonable to expect? What technical problems have researchers faced in developing imaging methodologies and what solutions are being developed in their ongoing studies? What, if any, imaging technique is developed to the point where it can be used in clinical practice?

In the area of neurolinguistics and neurobiological theory a number of advances can be expected in an improved understanding of the functional and morphological asymmetries or regions of the brain that have been implicated by current research on developmental dyslexia, attention deficit disorder, language/reading impaired children, autistic individuals, and other diagnostic categories that have some potential relationship to learning disabilities. In this area, several questions emerge that need additional research including: Which activation tasks have some functional specificity? Are specific brain patterns of symmetry or reversed asymmetry in the region of the plana or posterior cortex correlated with the dyslexia syndrome? How are these regions of interest best measured and is it possible to obtain reliable data such that future studies might productively advance brain-behavior theory? How might future studies more closely link deviations in neurolinguistic processes frequently found in dyslexic individuals with deviations in functional brain morphology? Do other forms of learning disability converge or diverge from this type of finding? Are these brain imaging methods a potential resource for reducing the heterogeneity found in the population(s) currently defined as learning disabled.

Additional topics that will be addressed by NICHD supported research during the next decade include establishing a classification system for conceptualizing, defining, and diagnosing learning disabilities that provides convergent and divergent validity for the co-morbidity between different types of LD (mathematics, speaking, listening, reading, and writing), attention deficit disorders (ADD, ADHD, and hyperactivity), conduct disorders, and the social aspects of learning disabilities. The search for behavioral, physiological, neurological, or anatomical anomalies that could mark subtypes of learning disabilities will be significantly advanced through the discoveries of genetic influences on components of reading and other academic skills, be they polygenic, single gene or chromosomal abnormalities linked to LD related phenotypes. A limited number of comparative studies of different intervention methods in teaching and treating well defined populations of dyslexic children will provide a basis for developing more effective interventions. Finally, new technological devices may be developed that substitute for diminished function of individuals with dyslexia or other learning disabilities.

SUMMARY

The magnitude of the number of individuals currently meeting any of the variety of accepted definitions of dyslexia and LD would seem to justify a continued effort by the NICHD to learn more about the nature of these disabilities. The implications of an improved understanding of dyslexia and other learning disabilities for the future are that with better classification systems, more homogeneous groups of individuals with LD can be studied for biological and behavioral markers. These indicators of a learning disorder could be used as risk factors for establishing early medical and behavioral interventions specifically designed to effectively ameliorate the disabilities of the children at risk for poor academic performance. The model of mental retardation is instructive. During the early decades of this century all mental retardation was attributed to either nature or nurture. Knowledge of specific etiologies was not to be found. Causation was attributed to mothers, diets, disease, and moral culpability, all without much concern for empirical data or even a generally accepted theoretical framework. Through the later half of the century, numerous scientific discoveries led to understanding different causes for different forms of mental retardation. The past decades have witnessed an astounding number of new categories of mental retardation, some with treatment protocols that are effective for specific etiologies. The great hope for those with dyslexia or other learning disabilities is that over the next decade, a variety of specific etiologies—some of biologic origin and others with sociobehavioral bases—will be found that are responsive to early intervention. By reducing the number of individuals who are receiving no treatment and developing educational interventions that are specific rather than generic, the lives of those with dyslexia or other learning disabilities will be improved. The scientists funded by the NICHD who describe their work in this book provide the best hope for making progress in this field. The NICHD funding of four program projects and three LDRCs marks the end of the beginning of efforts to develop a multidisciplinary approach to dyslexia and learning disabilities. The Orton Dyslexia Society conference where these chapters were presented offered a opportunity for the leaders of the program projects and LDRCs to share their expertise with each other and a group of concerned and informed parents, service providers, and other scientists. These efforts to improve a scientific approach for gaining an understanding of dyslexia are just beginning to bear the sweet fruit of discovery. The decade of the '90s should prove an exciting time for all of us interested in finding the keys to unlocking the abilities of those individuals we call dyslexic or learning disabled.

The editors express their appreciation for the quality of the chapters provided by the authors. The editorial guidance provided by Elinor Hartwig and her staff at York Press continue to be the essential factor in putting together significant books on the subject of dyslexia. Her patience has been much appreciated.

REFERENCES

Defining and Subtyping Dyslexia. 85-HD-10 *NIH Guide to Grants and Contracts, 14:* No. 5, April 26, 1985.

Gray, D. B. and Kavanagh, J. F. 1985. *Biobehavioral Measures of Dyslexia.* York Press: Parkton, MD.

Learning Disabilities: Multidisciplinary Research Centers. 88-HD/NS-1, *NIH Guide to Grants and Contracts 17:* No. 13, April 18, 1988.

Learning Disabilities: Multidisciplinary Research Center: Specialized Research Center Grant (P50). 90-HD-02, *NIH Guide to Grants and Contracts 19:* No. 3, January 19, 1990.

Chapter • 1

Neurobehavioral Definition of Dyslexia

Frank Wood, Rebecca Felton,
Lynn Flowers, and Cecile Naylor

It is a truism that definition in science ultimately requires a specification of the operations used to measure the concept being defined: anything less than this now classical standard of operational definition will ultimately be unserviceable in any sustained and productive scientific investigation. If dyslexia research is measured against this standard, it is undisputed that the field lacks this fundamental prerequisite: no specifiable operations have even been stated, much less agreed to. In such a situation it is as easy to decry the lack of definition as it is difficult to produce one: the problem is precisely that no consensual concepts of the term's meaning are available to guide the defining operations. In other words, we have not yet defined dyslexia because we have not yet understood it. Our problem is with the subject of the definitional statement, not its predicate.

Faced with that state of affairs, we immediately confront a troublesome circularity: the concept cannot be defined until it is understood, but how shall it be understood if there is no definition of "what" is being understood? For example, if we seek to discover adult outcomes of childhood dyslexia, we might select children who are reading poorly, and follow them into adulthood—but what does "reading poorly" mean? Standardized tests of reading assess a variety of skills ranging from pronouncing single words to answering content questions on a written paragraph. Which of them is the reading skill whose adult outcome is sought? A definition of childhood reading disability

Supported by USPHS Grant HD-21887 to Bowman Gray School of Medicine that emphasized one of these skills—say, single word pronunciation—would necessarily imply a judgment that it was the more critical skill for "true" dyslexia. It is common to give less weight to paragraph comprehension, on the grounds that many factors not directly related to "pure" reading can interfere with paragraph comprehension regardless of word pronunciation or identification skill. In this view, "true" dyslexia is a more narrowly circumscribed disorder, more serious because it disables even the basic word identification process upon which comprehension depends. Whatever the merit of this definition, it does imply a theory of dyslexia, and if the definition itself is controversial, then it is because the theory of dyslexia is controversial.

Traditional, theory-laden methods of escape from this circularity have tended to rely on two rather different strategies; appeal to simpler, "underlying" mechanisms (such as "phonemic awareness"), or appeal to a clinically recognizable syndrome or cluster of symptoms. Even momentary reflection reveals the pitfalls. The appeal to an "underlying mechanism" still begs the question how we shall know if a given individual has the disorder whose underlying mechanism is being sought. Any claim about a particular individual is always vulnerable to the counterclaim that "this individual really doesn't have dyslexia, anyway." On the other hand, the appeal to a clinical syndrome or pattern (as when a Supreme Court justice remarked about obscenity, "I don't know how to define it, but I know it when I see it") sinks the defining operations in a sea of subjectivity and starts the irreconcilable argument, "You may not call it dyslexia, but it really is, anyway."

Against such approaches that presume in advance that there is a theoretically "deeper" construct—either in the form of an underlying mechanism or a clinical syndrome—the major alternative is to describe only the "surface" behavior of impaired reading, without assuming any deeper constructs or intervening variables. In this approach, dyslexia is simply poor reading. Since the approach immediately sinks in a mire of uninteresting causes for poor reading (such as blindness), exclusionary criteria are inevitably stated. Such criteria, however, immediately beg the question of where to draw the line: there is little debate about excluding severe mental retardation—as in microcephaly—but much debate about whether general intelligence must actually be higher than reading skill (so that the reading can be said to be "discrepant" from intelligence).

The more important problem is that the decision about which exclusionary factors are appropriate is inherently guided by theories of underlying mechanism or of clinical pattern. For example, exclusion of cases with diagnosable psychopathology (such as attention deficit hyperactivity disorder [ADHD]) is equivalent to assuming separate underlying mechanisms for ADHD and dyslexia. Removing attention deficit from the defining characteristics of dyslexia would certainly seem to suggest a theoretical bias on the definition of dyslexia as "cognitive" rather than "attentional."

Thus, in this second type of circularity, the attempt to escape from theory-laden constructs that define dyslexia is nonetheless burdened with theoretical assumptions about constructs that are said to be excluded from the definition of dyslexia. Then, as the exclusions (what dyslexia is not) come into sharp focus, the implicit assumptions (about what dyslexia is) can no longer be hidden. The resolve to deal only with theory-neutral, surface behaviors cannot be kept.

Circularity, whether involving question-begging underlying mechanisms and clinical syndromes or involving theories implicit in exclusionary criteria, thus characterizes the current state of the art in the definition and understanding of dyslexia. The recourse for investigators of dyslexia should then be the same as that of explorers who find themselves circling in the wilderness: get to know the terrain better. More precisely, circling is a symptom of deficient acquaintance with the environment through which the path is sought. A map of the path in isolation is unhelpful: landmarks, off the path, are required.

On the other hand, in the same analogy, an exploring expedition by definition begins in ignorance and makes the maps as it goes. So, too, with science: a condition of definitional circularity and imprecision simply indicates the relatively early (and particularly interesting) phase of the inquiry. The serviceable operational definitions that characterize later stages of inquiry must await the successful completion of the initial exploratory, map-making phase. That is the context of the following studies: they represent a preliminary stage of investigating the question of defining dyslexia. As such, they may point the reader toward a clarification of definitional issues, particularly by showing the consequences of certain surface definitions. Thus, they may illustrate features of the landscape through which the path of definition ultimately can be constructed.

The studies reviewed here are part of an integrated program project funded by the National Institute of Child Health and Human Development for the specific purpose of defining and subtyping dyslexia.

STUDY 1: FIRST GRADE READING DISABILITY[1]

Sample and Method

A comprehensive series of neuropsychological and educational tests was administered to 485 children constituting a random sample of

---

[1]This study is reported in detail in the January, 1989, issue of the *Journal of Learning Disabilities*, by Felton and Wood.

first-grade children from the Winston-Salem/Forsyth County School System, in Winston-Salem, North Carolina. Their parents and teachers also were interviewed in an attempt to identify any of an extensive range of symptoms of attentional disorder and related forms of childhood psychopathology in the children.

A particular form of discrepancy definition of reading disability was employed. The Word Identification subtest of the Woodcock–Johnson Psychoeducational Battery (Woodcock and Johnson 1977) was employed as the single criterion measure of reading ability. It is a test of the ability to pronounce real words from print. The Peabody Picture Vocabulary Test (Dunn and Dunn 1981) was selected as the single "control" test, from which "discrepant" performance on the Word Identification subtest would be measured.

The rationale for this choice of the Peabody was that single word reading, on Woodcock–Johnson Word Identification, would be determined not only by actual ability to decode words from print (the criterion behavior) but also by basic knowledge of the words themselves (i.e., by vocabulary). A picture vocabulary test like the Peabody is particularly useful for assessing vocabulary, since no verbal response is required in the test. A Word Identification score sufficiently below the Peabody score would then represent a level of reading that was worse than what could be explained by poor vocabulary. To that extent, then, the deficit could be attributed to impaired decoding of words, "discrepant" from vocabulary, i.e., from the major non-reading skill that contributes to performance on the reading criterion.

Regression was employed to determine discrepancy between Woodcock–Johnson Word Identification and Peabody Picture Vocabulary. First, the multiple regression for predicting Word Identification from age, sex, and Peabody was calculated. That yielded a predicted Word Identification score, given an individual's age, sex, and Peabody score. This predicted score was then compared to the actual score, and a residual was obtained. These residuals were studentized and expressed as z-scores, representing the number of standard deviations away from the line of perfect prediction. Thus, percentiles can be assigned to the residuals, to represent the likelihood of obtaining a residual of a certain size.

Parenthetically, it is noteworthy that this type of prediction overcomes the simplistic but still common error of expecting the criterion (reading) to be as far from the mean (in standard deviations) as the predictor (vocabulary). That expectation is true only when the correlation between predictor and criterion is 1.0. In this case, the correlation being .85, a Peabody score of 70 with z-score of -2, for example, would predict a Word Identification score of 74 if expressed on a standard scale. That is a value that corresponds to a z-score that is .85 (the correlation) times the Peabody z-score. Thus, an individual with a reading standard score of 70 and a Peabody score of 70 would actually be reading somewhat worse than expected from the Peabody.

It is interesting that gender had no effect on the prediction of reading in this multiple regression—a point discussed more fully in the section entitled *Supplement to Study 1*, below.

From the above calculations, all cases whose discrepancy was at or below the fifth percentile were designated as the reading-disabled group. For comparison, a group of nondiscrepant readers was also assembled, composed of all subjects whose discrepancies ranged from the 16th to the 84th percentiles (−1 to +1 z-score for the discrepancy). The 5 to 16 percentile band (−2 to −1 z-score) was considered borderline, of uncertain degree of disability, hence excluded from the study. The 84 to 99 percentile band (greater than +1 z-score) was also excluded, so as to remove superior readers from the intended comparison between poor readers and average readers. These definitions yielded 25 poor readers and 333 average readers.

Two questions were of major interest to definitional issues in dyslexia: (1) whether there are reliable cognitive-neuropsychological test correlates of first grade reading test performance; and (2) if so, whether these correlates are separable from any cognitive correlates of ADHD.

Results and Discussion

The results are presented in detail in Felton and Wood (1989). For purposes of the present discussion, we may summarize them as showing that reading disability itself, distinct from the degree of ADHD, was statistically strongly related, at *p* values of less than .001, to tests of rapid naming (Denckla and Rudel 1976), confrontation naming (Kaplan, Goodglass, and Weintraub 1982), and phonemic awareness (Stanovich, Cunningham, and Cramer 1984). Other language, visuospatial, and memory tasks were unrelated to reading disability; and, whereas ADHD had some independent statistical effect on verbal memory and visual scanning tests, ADHD was unrelated to the naming and phonemic awareness tests that characterized reading disability itself. More importantly, there was no evidence of an interaction between ADHD and reading disability in determining or predicting cognitive test performance. In other words, ADHD and reading had separable cognitive effects, unrelated and noninteracting.

For purposes of the present discussion, it is particularly noteworthy that the reading-disabled children had significantly more teacher-reported ADHD symptoms than the non-reading-disabled children. If this is taken as evidence that ADHD is actually more common among reading-disabled children than among average readers, then an important potential confound in dyslexia research is illustrated: any comparison of reading-disabled to average-reading children, on tests of cognitive function, will be contaminated by the cognitive effects of ADHD. This potential brings us to the first of our three conclusions from this study:

1.   Any attempt to define dyslexia must deal with the ADHD problem. Only two options are really available: either consider ADHD an optional symptom within the clinical syndrome of dyslexia or consider ADHD as a separate disorder with separable cognitive consequences. The former is clinically appealing (since the clinical stereotype of dyslexia has often included attention deficit), but it sacrifices precision in the definition of the mechanism of disordered reading, since that mechanism is statistically separable from the ADHD mechanism of disordered attention.

On the other hand, if the second recourse is adopted, and reading disability is studied in isolation from ADHD symptoms, then another important theoretical possibility may be foreclosed: ADHD and reading disability may simply be slightly different manifestations of the same underlying pathophysiological process, differing perhaps only in the random placement of the congenital lesion. In particular, a genetic study might have to consider the possibility that either ADHD or dyslexia is the behavioral phenotype of a single genotype.

The best choice clearly would be a separate accounting of the cognitive correlates of reading disability and ADHD. This improves the description of underlying mechanisms and directs attention to particular, discrete neurobehavioral processes (largely linguistic ones, in the case of dyslexia). This choice must, however, explicitly reserve and leave open the possibility of a common pathophysiology for the two disorders. The clinical, pathophysiological "type" might not be synonymous with either "underlying mechanism."

2.   The demonstration that a particular subset of linguistic processes (naming and phonemic awareness) correlates with reading disability is limited to what might be termed "whole group" analyses. The demonstration suffices to identify the major cognitive correlates of reading disability only for the group as a whole (and, therefore, for a substantial majority of its members). It does not exclude the possibility, however, that relatively rare subtypes of reading disability exist with deficits other than linguistic: it only indicates that such subtypes, if they exist, are sufficiently rare as to have no measurable impact on the group differences between dyslexic and average readers.

It is important to consider the problem of demonstrating these rare subtypes. Cluster analysis is somewhat handicapped if the sought-after cluster is rare, since the signal/noise ratio (or ratio of true score variance to error variance, including measurement error) becomes unfavorable as the target cluster becomes relatively small. The recourse of even larger sample sizes naturally comes to mind, but a legitimate cost-benefit issue then arises: at what point is the proposed subtype sufficiently rare as to be not "worth" studying? The question may have one theoretically appealing answer when basic mechanisms, rare or common, are sought, but another practical answer in applied school settings where cost is an issue.

3. In this study the "discrepancy" definition that was employed left open an unresolved confound—whether the cognitive correlates of poor reading are due to the absolutely low level of reading itself, or due to the discrepancy with vocabulary. Because the discrepancy definition was rather stringent (requiring a reading score that is two standard deviations below the regression line for predicting reading from picture vocabulary), only a very few cases—indeed only two in the total sample of 25—had reading scores at or above the total sample mean. Thus, the data do not permit a definitive inference about whether it was absolute reading or discrepancy that was responsible for the cognitive correlates. Study 2 is a study of adults who had been dyslexic as children. In this study the absolute effects of reading level and IQ are accounted for separately by using a multivariate general linear model of analysis.

SUPPLEMENT TO STUDY 1: THE ROLE OF DEMOGRAPHIC
VARIABLES IN THE DEFINITION OF DYSLEXIA IN THE FIRST GRADE[2]

Gender is widely held to be critical in the phenotypic expression of the disability that constitutes dyslexia. Most studies of clinically ascertained cases show ratios of three or four to one, male to female, in dyslexic samples (see the thorough review of this entire question by Vogel [1990]). Few studies, however, have approached the question epidemiologically, thus bypassing whatever referral mechanisms are in place for identifying dyslexic children in the schools. Even if boys are far more common in referred and diagnosed dyslexic samples, the presence of a referral bias could obscure the true proportions of the disorder, by sex, in a normally distributed population. The sample in the above study, carefully constructed to represent a random cross-section of the first-grade population of the school system, permits a more direct test of this question. Once again, a variety of statistical approaches is possible, ranging from the imposition of a single-cut score below which all cases are considered dyslexic to the other extreme of simply

---

[2]These findings were *not* reported in the Felton and Wood (1989) study.

comparing the entire distributions across the range, for both boys and girls.

There is little ambiguity in the result, whatever statistical approach is used. In simple fact, there was no cut score of reading ability that could be used to define a dyslexic population whose gender ratio was at all different from that of the sample as a whole (53% male). No cut score established a dyslexic population whose proportion even approached being significantly different from the sample population. The other approach, in some ways a more comprehensive one, was to compare the two distributions of the male and female subsamples, to see if they differed statistically. The Kolgomorov–Smirnoff test—similar to a chi-square test—was used to compare the frequency distributions to see if they differ from the distribution that would be estimated from the sample as a whole. In this case, as well, nothing approaching a sigificant difference was demonstrated.

Accordingly, in contrast to the conventional stereotype, and consistent with the report by Shaywitz et al. (1990), we find no evidence of gender in the subject or the predicate of the definition of dyslexia. It is natural to suspect a referral bias, but the details of that bias are not at all clear from the available data: it is certainly possible, as Shaywitz et al. (1990) have suggested, that temperament differences between boys and girls cause boys to be more noticeable to their teachers, and consequently more often referred. More importantly, perhaps, we do not know if this equality of the sexes will be maintained in later grades, until the full follow-up studies are done. Thus, the findings—while unexpected—raise a host of additional questions. For purposes of our present discussion, however, they do call into question any role of gender in any aspect of the definition of dyslexia.

The effect of race was more complicated. In the above sample of 485 first graders, race had no significant predictive effect on reading scores, once vocabulary scores (from the Peabody) were accounted for in the prediction equation. In other words, consistent with the conventional expectation, once we knew a child's vocabulary and age, we gained no additional predictive power from knowing the child's race, so far as the prediction of first-grade reading scores was concerned.

Data are available, however, on the third grade individual testing for this sample. Three hundred fifty of the children took the Woodcock–Johnson in the spring of their third-grade year, approximately two years after the above reported first-grade testing. The disconcerting fact about these third-grade follow-up data was simply this: race was a significant predictor, at $p = .001$, of the third grade Woodcock–Johnson reading score, even when the most powerful predictor (first grade Woodcock–Johnson reading score) was also in the equation. In other words, some additional predictive power, for predicting third-grade Woodcock–Johnson reading scale score for age, is obtained from knowing a child's race—even if the child's first-grade reading score is also known. To put it yet another way, if children are statistically equated for first-grade reading score, still there is a race effect for predicting third-grade reading.

An analysis of the distributions of first-grade reading scores establishes that a floor effect is highly unlikely to be the explanation for the absence of race effect in the first grade. Even children scoring well off the floor in the first grade show the same race effect by the third grade. We also tested a variety of other demographic variables in the prediction equation and found them unable to account for the result. Thus, parental marital status (single or married), parental education, parental status as a welfare recipient, and even the number of books estimated by the parent to be present in the home (or the number of newspaper and magazine subscriptions) all had no effect, whether singly or in combination. The presence of any or all of these additional variables in the prediction equation did not remove the race effect from its potency as an independent predictor of third-grade reading.

It is natural, since parent socioeconomic variables were unrelated to the effect, to expect once again the operation of some kind of systemic bias, perhaps from teachers or others—in its own way, similar to the above described possibility of a referral bias for boys. No data of any kind, however, are available to confirm the possibility of a bias within the educational system itself—and we caution against jumping to that conclusion. Instead, we should ask the larger question of whether there is anything about the educational or cultural situation of minority-race children that works to their disadvantage after first grade. (The other way of asking the question would be: what is the difference between the cultural and educational experience of minority-race children before first grade and after first grade, so that only the experience after first grade works to their disadvantage?)

From the perspective of the problem of defining dyslexia as a neurobehavioral construct, the above two demographic issues are important chiefly because they can complicate efforts to obtain a culture-free definition. On the one hand, it appears that some sort of strong sex bias operates to skew the distribution of males and females, and thus superficially obscure the possibility of equal sex ratios in the population as a whole. By contrast, the race findings suggest some sort of bias or disadvantage that shows up not in referral patterns for the identification of clinical cases of dyslexia but in standardized test scores themselves, after first grade. Here are two examples, then, of the potentially confusing and complicating role of demographic and cultural variables. In principle, the role of such variables cannot be overlooked in the quest for accurate definitions of dyslexia itself.

STUDY 2: THE ADULT NEUROPSYCHOLOGICAL
PHENOTYPE OF CHILDHOOD DYSLEXIA[3]

Sample and Method

This study focuses on a group of adults, previously evaluated in childhood, whose childhood records have been preserved for research purposes in the June Lyday and Samuel T. Orton Collection of the Columbia University Libraries. Included in this group are individuals who were reading disabled as children as well as those who were evaluated for other reasons (including benign ones) and who showed no evidence of reading disabilities. From these records, it is possible to consider the relationship of reading ability in childhood to cognitive skills in adulthood—a relationship that can be separated from the attainment of adult reading skills.

The study sample consisted of 115 adults, ranging from 20.2 to 44.6 years of age (M = 33.1 years). They had initially been evaluated between 1957 and 1972 by June Lyday Orton, and childhood intelligence and achievement test scores were available in the Orton Collection. There were 18 females and 97 males—all free of any history of neurological impairment such as head trauma or seizures and free of current major psychopathology on the Schedule for Affective Disorders and Schizophrenia, Lifetime Version (Endicott and Spitzer 1978).

Childhood intelligence scores consisted mostly of the age-appropriate Wechsler Intelligence Test scores. However, for the six cases where Wechsler scores were unavailable, Stanford Binet, California Short Form, or Slossen IQ's were substituted. Scores from the Gray Oral Reading Paragraphs Test (GORT) (Gray 1955) and reading subtest of the Wide Range Achievement Test (WRAT) (Jastak and Bijou 1946) were also available on most cases; however, the IOTA Word Test (Monroe 1932) or Gilmore Oral Reading Test (Gilmore 1951) replaced missing WRAT or GORT scores.

To be classified as reading disabled (RD) in this study, subjects were required to have reading quotients (Reading Age × 100/Chronological Age) of less than or equal to 82 on both the GORT and the WRAT or their equivalents; non-reading-disabled (NRD) subjects had to have greater than 91 on both tests; and all other combinations of scores were classified as borderline (BL). This avoids an extreme-groups approach that eliminates borderline cases (see Pennington [1986]; and Share et al. [1987]). Moreover, the requirement for impairment on two separate tests was intended to protect against false posi-

---

[3]This study is reported in detail in *Brain and Language,* in press, by Felton, Naylor, and Wood.

tives on a single test while at the same time broadening the concept of impaired reading to include paragraph text as well as single words (Rudel 1985). This particular cut score of 82 is the equivalent of being one and one half years behind in the third grade, or two years behind in the sixth grade. The requirement for this level of deficit on both tests is estimated to include less than five percent of the normal population.

As indicated above, the definition of reading disability did not include a discrepancy from IQ (or any other ability measure). Although several studies (e.g., Siegel [1989] and Share et al. [1987]) have not found meaningful differences between poor readers whose IQ is consonant with their reading and poor readers whose IQ is discrepant (on the high side) from their reading, this remains in principle a research question. (See also Satz and Van Nostrand [1973]; Satz et al. [1978].) The strategy in this study was to assess the impact of IQ as a separate source of variance, distinct from reading level as operationalized above. This is equivalent to the use of IQ as a covariate, except that the intent is to quantify the predictive power of both sources of variance separately.

Included in the test battery was a battery of neuropsychological tests to determine the adult cognitive phenotype in developmental dyslexia. This group of tests included not only the Wechsler Adult Intelligence Scale–Revised (WAIS–R) (Wechsler 1981), but a series of specific tests of phonemic awareness, naming, visuo-spatial skills, and memory.

Results

The adult neuropsychological test scores were z-standardized to an independent sample of 23 normal control subjects who matched the subjects in age ($M = 31.2$), education ($M = 16.3$), and Wechsler IQ (108.2). These subjects had average adult reading scores: mean raw score of 84.3 on the GORT; and mean standard scores of 104.8, 101.3, and 102.1, respectively, on the WRAT reading, spelling, and arithmetic subtests.

Though not significantly different from NRD at the time of adult testing, the RD were significantly older than NRD (but not significantly higher in grade placement) at the time of their childhood evaluation. These differences due to age at initial evaluation were controlled by covariance in the subsequent analyses.

A general linear model (essentially a multivariate analysis of covariance with unequal Ns) tested the prediction of adult neuropsychological data from the childhood reading level and IQ, with socioeconomic status (SES) as a covariate in the model.

In absolute terms, the RD group performed consistently worse than the other two groups on most neuropsychological tests including tests of memory, visual perceptual processing, visuomotor speed, and mental flexibility. However, separate univariate analyses revealed that few of these differences were related to a history of reading disability after differences in childhood intelligence and SES were accounted for.

On the other hand, tests of rapid naming and nonword reading (word attack) were significantly different, despite covariance for preexisting differences in childhood intelligence and SES.

Given that adult educational attainment or intelligence may have affected performance on these adult neuropsychological measures, the data were also analyzed with adult IQ and educational level controlled. Rapid naming and nonword reading remained significant and a test of phoneme manipulation (Lindamood and Lindamood 1971) was then also significant at $p < .01$.

Discussion

These results are similar to our childhood findings (Study 1, above) and to other adult studies (Decker 1989; Bruck 1989). The Decker (1989) study showed the best discriminators of adult reading disability to be speed of letter naming and speed of recognition of pronounceable nonwords; and the Bruck (1989) study also showed that extreme difficulty in reading nonwords (based on accuracy and latency data) characterized adult dyslexics.

The consistent and instructive feature of all these studies is the persistence into adulthood of a phonemically related processing deficit. Given a reading disability defined from childhood reading performance, the studies show this persisting deficit regardless of actual improvements in reading as measured in adulthood. The similarities between the reading-related cognitive deficits in childhood (Felton and Brown in press) and those in adulthood are striking.

These results support current models of reading disability that implicate phonological processing as the critical domain of dyslexic impairment (Jorm et al. 1983; Pennington et al. 1987; Stanovich 1988). Most often, deficits in phonological awareness have been emphasized; but our data here suggest that phonological recoding in word retrieval, as in rapid naming, is also a salient feature. We note, furthermore (Felton and Wood 1989; Felton and Brown 1990), that rapid naming and phonological awareness are not necessarily correlated and could constitute separate aspects of the overall phonological processing deficit in dyslexia. (See also Ellis and Miles [1981] and Perfetti's verbal efficiency theory [1985] for discussions about the salience of lexical access and word retrieval as central processes in reading.)

For purposes of the discussion about definition that is the focus of this chapter, the above study is of particular interest for the following reasons:

1. This study separates the effect of IQ from those of reading disability (both factors measured in childhood). The typical general linear model permits separate accounting of the variance in adult cognitive test scores, explainable from reading and IQ. Notwithstanding this difference from Study 1 (in which a discrepancy definition was used), a highly similar result is obtained. The implication might then be justified, that phonological processing deficit—including its word retrieval component—is a correlate of reading disability in isolation, distinct from IQ and regardless of whether discrepant from IQ or not.

By accounting separately for IQ and reading, the study tends to focus attention more in the direction of underlying mechanisms or processes (here, reading in isolation) and away from clinical syndromes. It may be that such a focus is inherent in the statistical approach itself, since the approach assumes the separable operation of different variables—or at least their separate correlated variances—even within a single case.

2. Consistent with the trend of the study toward a process rather than a syndromic definition, the study establishes a borderline (and therefore ambiguous) level of severity of reading deficit. The more one focuses on process, the more difficult it becomes to draw the line, in individual cases, between those who "have" the process and those who do not (or are truly deficient in the process). While this is not at all disconcerting to the more cognitively oriented researcher, it does cut somewhat against the grain of clinical sensibilities, since it does not provide a crisp clinical marker for affected and unaffected cases.

3. It is reassuring that the adult phenotype is so similar to the child phenotype, even when absolute rather than discrepancy definitions of dyslexia are used. The persistence of these phenotypic cognitive markers of phonemic processing and rapid naming deficits, all the way into adulthood, does give strong impetus to the concept of a persisting, constitutional deficit. Investigations about the neuroanatomical aspects of the "underlying mechanism" of the deficit—whether process or syndromic—is then the natural focus of the following study.

STUDY 3: ADULT FUNCTIONAL NEUROIMAGING
PHENOTYPE OF CHILDHOOD DYSLEXIA[4]

Introduction, Sample, and Method

The above studies implicate persistent language deficits and raise the question of a left hemisphere anatomical substrate. The possibility of

---

[4]This study is reported in detail in *Archives of Neurology,* in press, by Flowers, Wood, and Naylor.

anomalous organization of the left hemisphere in dyslexic individuals arises from two different sources.

1. Post-mortem has demonstrated cytoarchitectural anomalies— somewhat though not exclusively concentrated in the left peri-Sylvian area—in dyslexic brains (Kaufman and Galaburda 1989; Galaburda et al. 1985; Duane 1989). These abnormalities are thought to occur during the wave of cell migration that forms the upper cortical layers. Animal models can simulate these abnormalities by the placement of small lesions in the immature cortex: these lesions then alter the migration of cells into the superficial cortical layers (Dvorak, Feit, and Jurankova 1978). In humans, a specific etiology for such lesions has not been proven, but slower maturation of the left hemisphere is thought to render it more vulnerable (than the right hemisphere) to these anomalies (Geschwind and Galaburda 1985).

2. Altered macroneural organization in reading-disabled subjects is suggested by the absence of the normal left-greater-than-right asymmetry in the posterior temporal planum (Tp) in autopsy material (Kaufmann and Galaburda 1989; Galaburda et al. 1985) and in computerized tomography and magnetic resonance imaging (Hier et al. 1978; Rumsey et al. 1986). Anomalous cell migration is a possible etiology for these changes as well; for example, after creation of a unilateral frontal lesion in the fetal monkey, larger than normal occipital cortices are found bilaterally (Goldman 1978; Goldman-Rakic and Rakic 1984). Abnormally reduced cell death (or "pruning"), possibly from lack of normal competition during cortico-genesis, is implicated. Applied to reading disability, this logic suggests that symmetrical temporal plana also could result from an original unilateral lesion.

Physiological evidence also implicates atypical functional organization of the left hemisphere. Ojemann's (1983) intraoperative brain electrical stimulation studies are particularly relevant. They show that sites functionally involved with core language skills (for instance, naming, orofacial sequencing, and phonetic discrimination) are normally distributed closely along both banks of the Sylvian fissure (Ojemann 1983; Ojemann and Whitaker 1978). However, there was marked redistribution of these functions in some left hemisphere dominant epileptic patients: males with lower verbal IQs (below 90) showed a posterior displacement of naming-related sites (away from the superior temporal gyrus and toward the angular gyrus). Ojemann and Whitaker (1978) reported also a particular association between early left anterior temporal lesions and a wider distribution of naming sites in the posterior temporal and parietal cortex. Rasmussen and Milner (1977) have proposed a similar association between early lesions encroaching on the temporal language areas and a displacement to parietal cortex. (See also the non-human primate studies of Glees and Cole [1950] and Cole and Glees [1954].)

The 133-Xenon regional cerebral blood flow (rCBF) method is particularly well suited for monitoring the macro-neural correlates of language activation: the temporal resolution permits a task lasting only a few minutes; the relative safety and low cost allow the use of large normal reference groups and multiple conditions (Wood 1980, 1983); and resolution of the gray versus white matter flow exceeds that of other methods.

We predicted that: (1) in normals, a task requiring the processing of auditory verbal stimuli would be accompanied by focal activation of the left hemisphere perisylvian (superior temporal) regions; and (2) in a comparison of adult dyslexics to adult normal readers (defined in both cases by childhood scores), there would be displacement or spread of activation in dyslexic readers from the temporal to the posterior temporo-parietal regions.

Two separate samples were studied with the 133-Xenon method: the first involved the concurrent correlation of orthographic task accuracy with blood flow during the task, in healthy adults with no history of reading problems. The second sample permitted two analyses: (a) a replication of the above correlation within a group of adults that are sub-classified by their documented childhood reading scores; and (b) a prediction, directly from childhood reading levels, of adult blood flow independent of task accuracy.

For the first study, 69 subjects (39 males and 30 females) underwent rCBF measurement during performance of an auditory orthographic analysis task. They were all right-handed and reported no history of reading difficulties or repeating grades in school. The 83 subjects (72 males and 11 females) in the second sample were a subset of the Orton sample described in Study 2 of this chapter, above. All subjects had both childhood and adulthood IQ scores of at least 80 on either the verbal or performance scale.

Assignment to childhood reading levels was as described above in Study 2 of this chapter: Boder reading quotients (over age alone, Boder and Jarrico 1982) had to be less than or equal to 82 on both the WRAT Reading (Jastak and Bijou 1946) and Gray Oral Reading (Gray 1955) tests in childhood, in order to yield a classification of reading disabled (RD). Both had to be above 91 to obtain a classification of non-reading disabled (NRD); all others were classified as borderline (BL). By this rule, 33 were RD; 27 were BL; and 23 were NRD. All were free of pulmonary dysfunction (for safety's sake in rCBF studies with inhalation). Seven were left-handed; six were ambidextrous (Briggs and Nebes 1975).

Regional cerebral blood flow was measured by a Novo Cerebrograph 32C system (Novo Diagnostic Systems, Bagsvaerd, Denmark), supported by a PDP-11 minicomputer for on-line monitoring of the technical quality of ongoing measurements. Risberg's Initial Slope Index (ISI), a relatively conservative index of gray matter activity (Prohovnik, Knudson, and Risberg 1985), was the dependent measure.

The orthographic analysis task, conducted during the rCBF measurement, required subjects to listen to common concrete nouns—occuring one every 2.5 seconds—and signal with a bilateral finger lift response if the word was exactly four letters long. A random half of the words met the target criterion. Task accuracy was calculated as signal detection accuracy or d-prime (Green and Swets 1966), to incorporate both the Hit and False Alarm rates and avoid response bias confounds.

Results and Discussion

Following common practice, each of the 16 ISI values obtained from each subject was expressed as a percent of hemispheric mean flow: (ISI/mean flow) × 100. These dependent measures were then predicted from task accuracy (the first two analyses) or childhood reading level (the third analysis), using a general linear model which included as covariates IQ, age, gender, and task order (since other tasks not related to the present study were used, in counterbalanced order). For the known effects of these covariates, see Naritomi et al. (1979); Hannay et al. (1983); Risberg, Maximilian, and Prohovnik (1977); and Wood et al. (1980). The two peri-Sylvian sites of interest were the inferior premotor area of Broca and the superior posterior temporal area of Wernicke. The angular gyrus region was expected from the Ojemann (1983) studies to be the site of displaced functional activity in language-deficient, reading-disabled subjects.

Experiment 1: Left hemisphere blood flow predicted by spelling task accuracy in 69 adults with no history of reading problems. In the general linear model, accuracy of task performance predicted blood flow in these normals only at left Wernicke's area but not at left Broca's area or at any other site. The prediction was independent of IQ, gender, age, or task order; and in a subset of 47 subjects on whom state anxiety measures were taken (Spielberger et al. 1983), statistical control for state anxiety also did not change the prediction of blood flow from task accuracy.

Thus, in this normal subject group, accuracy on a spelling-related task was related to focal activation of one left perisylvian region, Wernicke's area.

Experiment 2, Analysis A: Replication of the relationship between task accuracy and left hemisphere blood flow in subjects with widely varying, archivally documented childhood reading ability. Task performance again significantly predicted flow only at left Wernicke's area, independent of age, IQ, gender, and task order. Separate analyses found no effect of years of education, state anxiety, or handedness on the prediction of left temporal flow from task accuracy. This replication gives confidence that the proposed relationship of language activation to the left temporal area is a reliable one.

Experiment 2, Analysis B: Early reading ability as a predictor of cortical activation. The general linear model showed that good versus poor childhood readers differed significantly at the Wernicke's area site. That is not surprising, however, since poor readers performed the task less well, and task performance has been shown in both samples (69 normals and 83 Ortons) to predict left temporal flow. When task accuracy is entered as a covariate, then, the group differences in Wernicke's flow were abolished as would be expected.

The hypothesis was, however, that persons with reading disabilities would show not only less activation in the left temporal area, but a displacement of activation to a more posterior site, the angular gyrus. As predicted, the general linear model showed a significant inverse relationship between childhood reading level and flow (the RD group had higher flow than either the BL or NRD groups). Angular gyrus flow was higher in the RD group. Neither childhood verbal nor performance IQ, education, age, gender, state anxiety, or task order had any effect on this prediction.

Of special importance is the fact that this inverse relationship between childhood reading and angular gyrus activity is independent of task performance: even when accuracy of task performance is entered into the general linear model, the relationship holds strong at $p < .02$.

The high temporo-parietal flow of the RD group is also independent of adult reading improvement, as classified by the same two oral reading tests used to assign subjects to a childhood reading level.

Strictly speaking, then, the excess angular gyrus activation in dyslexic individuals is difficult to interpret as a pure displacement from the temporal activation that characterizes normal individuals: if it were, then it also would be expected to be correlated with task accuracy and with adult reading outcome.

What, then, is the proper explanation? Differential verbal experience—between dyslexic and normal individuals—is certainly one theoretical possibility: it is conceivable that lifelong dyslexia induces impoverished verbal experience, and that is what shows up in the flow differences. The lack of any covarying relationship of education to the flow differences, however, at least weakens this possibility.

Alternatively, it is a known phenomenon in functional neuroimaging research that the additional effort expended by subjects who perform poorly could be the explanation for the excess activation (see Wood 1990). Indeed, in this study, subject ratings of task difficulty were positively related to task performance at $r = .59$. However, task performance and self-reported task difficulty are both statistically independent of the relationship between reading impairment and angular gyrus activation.

Strategy differences between dyslexic and normal readers are also possible. They could, in principle, arise from inadequacies in the functioning of the left temporal cortex, thus precipitating or even forcing a *non-temporal*, perhaps a less auditorally related, strategy that is compatible with angular gyrus activation. This alternative angular gyrus strategy might be less efficient and ordinarily inhibited by good readers—hence the inverse relationship. That would imply a theory of dual, parallel pathways for the analysis of orthographic features of auditorally presented words—perhaps at a stage subsequent to the direct auditory–linguistic analysis ordinarily expected to occur in the auditory cortex. The preferred *temporal lobe* strategy for this later-stage orthographic processing might be more bound to the auditory signal, whereas the less efficient angular gyrus strategy might depend on an analysis of a visual image of the word. Still, it is difficult to understand why task accuracy or adult reading outcome would not be proportional to the tendency to invoke this alternate angular gyrus strategy. Nonetheless, if the strategy is indeed inefficient, then it would be at least theoretically possible for the angular gyrus activation to be statistically uncoupled from task performance or reading outcome.

It is finally possible that the congenital lesions presumed to occur in dyslexic individuals could induce a pattern of altered connectivity, in which axons normally targeted for the superior temporal region are instead relocated to targets near the angular gyrus. An example is found in studies of neonatal hamsters, where simultaneously lesioning visual target areas as well as auditory or somatosensory afferents results in visually driven synapses at auditory or somatosensory sites. (See Sur, Garraghty, and Roe 1988; Frost 1988.) In dyslexic individuals, a posterior relocation of embryonic axons would constitute a true structural displacement, established prenatally and remaining fixed. So formed, these atypical circuits perhaps would not be as efficient as those established under non-lesion conditions and would explain why fully normal functions would not develop.

However, a structural displacement model must also be qualified by the fact of uncoupling of angular gyrus activation from task accuracy and reading outcome. Similar to the case of strategy differences, the hypothesis would have to be that only a partial subset of functions are displaced, and these would have to be either quantitatively unrelated to task performance (as in "on–off" processors) or inefficient, so that task performance is only poorly related to angular gyrus activation.

Compensation must also be considered. About half of the individuals with reading disabilities have essentially normal WRAT–R Reading and Gray Oral Reading test scores in adulthood. Perhaps they do have alternative compensatory pathways, or perhaps they overpractice their existing but initially deficient pathways (Bradley and Bryant 1983). Our data show no correlates of such compensation, however: these methods, so far, have been inadequate to detect compensatory mechanisms, despite the 25 year longitudinal timespan between childhood and adulthood reading.

Indeed, cortical compensatory mechanisms in humans have in general escaped clear detection, although near-normal language skills can develop in spite of early left hemisphere lesions including hemispherectomy itself (Dennis and Whitaker 1976).

This physiological study carries the general trend of the studies reviewed in this chapter even further in the direction of an underlying mechanism or process. Given the particular results, it also provides an instructive general commentary on the question of defining dyslexia, in the following particular ways.

1. As would be necessary in any credible study of a supposedly abnormal physiological mechanism, the first prerequisite is to define the normal mechanism. This study, accordingly, establishes that left temporal blood flow during an orthographic task performance is positively correlated with accuracy of performance on that task. There are, in principle, several ways to isolate a normal mechanism using physiological measures during cognitive task performance. For example, another common approach is to consider change from baseline (some relatively neutral, supposedly "non-activated" state). The task in question, in this particular method, is then identified with those regions that become more active during task performance than during the control or rest state. That approach was not chosen in this study, however, because the focus was on individual differences in task performance, differences that are obscured by the baseline control method.

In the present study, the individual differences—even in normal individuals—in task performance were taken as the basic indicator of activation. That is an assumption that is always arguable, but it is nonetheless one that more naturally sets the stage for subsequent study of an impaired group (as was done in this case).

2. The identification of the left temporal locus as critical to task performance is, of course, greatly strengthened by its replication in a second large sample. This allows the individual difference in left temporal activation to be correlated with differences in childhood reading

level, apart from childhood IQ and certain other control variables (age, sex, state anxiety, and the like). In terms of the definitional questions at stake in this chapter, the approach is particularly interesting, inasmuch as it allows first the normal variation to be localized in the brain. This localization is then followed by a demonstration that a substantial portion of that normal variation is predictable from childhood reading independent of adult outcome.

Research programs aimed at processes or underlying mechanisms must inevitably confront this very issue: is the alleged underlying process a normal process that is simply absent, or is it actually an abnormal process itself? If only experiments 1 and 2A of this physiological study are considered, the implication would be only that a normal process is absent or reduced in amplitude in dyslexia. In other words, the orthographic analysis task ordinarily invokes left temporal activation; dyslexic individuals are deficient at orthographic task performance; and, consequently, dyslexic individuals are deficient in left temporal lobe activation. This conclusion, however, if standing alone, would also fall victim to another of the contentious circularities that bedevil dyslexia research: the left temporal lobe activation failure might be a consequence instead of a cause of the deficient task performance in dyslexic individuals. Fortunately, we partly escape this fate by the results of experiment 2B, showing evidence of the positive presence of an otherwise suppressed process, in addition to evidence of a deficient process. It is difficult to attribute this abnormality to a consequence rather than a cause of dyslexia, since it is better predicted by childhood reading than by adulthood reading outcome.

3.   The finding of abnormal, excessive left temporoparietal or angular gyrus activation in dyslexia thus advances the agenda of discovering the underlying mechanism—not simply the underlying mechanism of reading itself, but the particular mechanism of abnormal performance. From the perspective of definitional issues, this is particularly interesting because the abnormal case (childhood reading disability) is not simply an extreme on the normal distribution, but instead a case showing features either suppressed or not present in the normal population at all. Oddly, this finding somewhat balances the debate between underlying process and clinical syndrome, since it does suggest a truly different "type" that can be defined or marked by this abnormal focus of excess activation.

CONCLUDING COMMENTS

If all the above three studies are considered in sequence, then they can be said to begin by pointing strongly in the direction of underlying process and away from the notion of a clinical syndrome as the better approach to defining dyslexia. The separation of cognitive effects of ADHD from those of reading disability alone, and the long-term salience of phonemic deficits in childhood as well as adulthood phenotypes of reading disability are clearly supportive of a mechanistic association between reading and phonological processing—across the range of impaired to normal reading. Curiously, however, as the sequence proceeds to a neurophysiological level in Study 3, it reinstates the importance of typology—here seen as a distinct, non-normal process of angular gyrus activation that is present in dyslexic individuals and not in normal individuals. In pursuing the impaired phonological process or mechanism to a cerebral level of analysis, we are once again found to have circled back to the starting point of typology.

Nonetheless, consistent with the introductory arguments of this chapter, we can find the circularity instructive—in this case, it has at least proceeded beyond the behavioral domain to incorporate physiological processes at the macro-neural level. Perhaps with higher resolution techniques, then, we can expect to proceed once more toward a process definition, this time at the physiological level. The experience of this review might then lead us to predict yet another typology—perhaps at the micro-neural or even at the genetic level. Though circular in some senses, this would nevertheless represent progress through successive levels of analysis. Certain features of this landscape may already be considered instructive, and can be summarized as the following simple propositions.

1. Case definition of reading disability is often confounded, at least in childhood, by attention deficit disorder—whose separate cognitive correlates should be removed from consideration.

2. In a way that is conceptually similar to the ADHD confound, IQ or other general ability measures including vocabulary can be separated from reading disability itself. Discrepancy formulae are not the only way to accomplish this, nor even the statistically best way. It appears that the isolation of reading alone, and the separate accounting for IQ effects, can both be accomplished by statistical multivariate approaches that assess the separate variance accounted for by each variable.

3. Gender, race, and other demographic and cultural variables need careful attention, since they may operate to confuse the definition of cases.

4. Whatever definition is proposed for dyslexia should be demonstrably persistent over time—even from first grade through adulthood.

5. Physiological definitions may ultimately provide surprising new support for clinical typology definitions, even while they are at the

same time clarifying proposed underlying processes. Accordingly, it is premature to foreclose either approach. Underlying process and clinical typology should both be studied at the current stage of research in dyslexia.

REFERENCES

Boder, E., and Jarrico, S. 1982. *The Boder Test of Reading–Spelling Patterns: A Diagnostic Screening Test for Subtypes of Reading Disability.* New York: Grune and Stratton.

Bradley, L., and Bryant, P. 1983. Categorizing sounds and learning to read: A causal connection. *Nature* 302:419–21.

Brigg, G. G., and Nebes, R. D. 1975. Patterns of hand preference in a student population. *Cortex* 11:230–38.

Bruck, M. 1989. Word recognition skills of adults with childhood diagnoses of dyslexia. *Developmental Psychology* 26:439–54.

Cole, J., and Glees, P. 1954. Effects of small lesions in sensory cortex in trained monkeys. *Journal of Neurophysiology* 17:1–21.

Decker, S. 1989. Cognitive processing rates among disabled and normal reading young adults: A nine year follow-up study. *Reading and Writing: An Interdisciplinary Journal* 2:123–34.

Denckla, M. A., and Rudel, R. G. 1976. Naming of object drawings by dyslexic and other learning disabled children. *Brain and Language* 3:1–16.

Dennis, M., and Whitaker, H. A. 1976. Language acquisition following hemidecortication: Linguistic superiority of the left over the right hemisphere. *Brain and Language* 3:404–33.

Duane, D. D. 1989. Commentary on dyslexia and neurodevelopmental pathology. *Journal of Learning Disabilities* 22:219–20.

Dvorak, K., Feit, J., and Jurankova, Z. 1978. Experimentally induced focal microgyria and status varrucosus deformis in rats. *Acta Neuropathol* 44:121–29.

Dunn, L. D., and Dunn, L. M. 1981. *Peabody Picture Vocabulary Test–Revised.* Circle Pines, MN: American Guidance Service.

Ellis, N., and Miles, T. 1981. A lexical encoding deficiency. I. Experimental evidence. In *Dyslexia Research and Its Applications to Education,* eds. G. T. Pavlidis and T. R. Miles. Chichester, England: Wiley.

Endicott, J., and Spitzer, R. L. 1978. A diagnostic interview: The schedule for affective disorders and schizophrenia. *Archives of General Psychiatry* 35:837–44.

Felton, R. H., and Brown, I. S. 1990. Phonological processes as predictors of specific reading skills in children at risk for reading failure. *Reading and Writing: An Interdisciplinary Journal* 2:39–59.

Felton, R. H., and Brown, I. B. in press. Neuropsychological prediction of reading disabilities. In *Neuropsychological Foundations of Learning Disabilities: A Handbook of Issues, Methods, and Practice,* eds. J. E. Obrzut and G. W. Hynd. Orlando, FL: Academic Press.

Felton, R. H., and Wood, F. B. 1989. Cognitive deficits in reading disability and attention deficit disorder. *Journal of Learning Disabilities* 1:3–13.

Felton, R. H., Naylor, C. E., and Wood, F. B. in press. The neuropsychological profile of adult dyslexics. *Brain and Language.*

Flowers, D. L., Wood, F. B., and Naylor, C. E. in press. Regional cerebral blood flow correlates of language processes in adult dyslexics. *Archives of Neurology.*

Frost, D. D. 1988. Mechanisms of structural and functional development in the thalamus: Retinal projections to the auditory and somatosensory systems in normal and experimentally manipulated hamsters. In *Cellular Thalamic Mechanisms*, eds. M. Bentivoglio and R. Spreafico. Amsterdam: Elsevier Scientific Publishing Co.

Galaburda, A. M., Sherman, G. F., Rosen, G. D., Aboitiz, F., and Geschwind, N. 1985. Developmental dyslexia: Four consecutive patients with cortical anomalies. *Annals of Neurology* 18:222–33.

Geschwind, N., and Galaburda, A. M. 1985a, b, c. Cerebral lateralization: Biological mechanisms, associations, and pathology. *Archives of Neurology* 42: I(a)428–59, II(b)521–52, III(c)634–54.

Gilmore, J. V. 1951. *Gilmore Oral Reading Test.* New York: Harcourt, Brace and World, Inc.

Glees, P., and Cole, J. 1950. Recovery of skilled motor functions after small repeated lesions of motor cortex in macaque. *Journal of Neurophysiology* 13:137–48.

Goldman, P. S. 1978. Neuronal plasticity in primate telencephalon: Anomalous projections induced by prenatal removal of frontal cortex. *Science* 202:768–70.

Goldman-Rakic, P. S., and Rakic, P. 1984. Experimentally modified convolutional patterns in non-human primates: Possible relevance of connections to cerebral dominance in humans. In *Biological Foundation of Cerebral Dominance*, eds. N. Geschwind and A. M. Galaburda. Cambridge, MA: Harvard University Press.

Gray, W. S. 1955. *Standardized Oral Reading Paragraphs.* Indianapolis: Bobbs-Merrill.

Green, D. M., and Swets, J. 1966. *Signal Detection Theory.* New York: Wiley Press.

Hannay, H. J., Leli, D. A., Falgout, J. C., Katholi, C. R., and Halsey, J. H. 1983. rCBF for middle-aged males and females during right-left discrimination. *Cortex* 19:465–74.

Hier, D. B., LeMay, M., Rosenberger, P. B., and Perlo, V. P. 1978. Developmental dyslexia: Evidence for a subgroup with a reversal of cerebral asymmetry. *Archives of Neurology* 35:90–92.

Jastak, J., and Bijou, S. 1946. *Wide Range Achievement Test.* Wilmington: Jastak Associates.

Jorm, A. F. 1983. Specific reading retardation and working memory: A review. *British Journal of Psychology* 74:311–42.

Kaplan, E., Goodglass, H., and Weintraub, S. 1982. *Boston Naming Test.* Philadelphia: Lea & Febiger.

Kaufman, W. E., and Galaburda, A. M. 1989. Cerebrocortical microdysgenesis in neurologically normal subjects: A histopathologic study. *Neurology* 39:238–44.

Lindamood, C. H., and Lindamood, P. C. 1971. *Lindamood Auditory Conceptualization Test.* Boston: Teaching Resources Corporation.

Monroe, M. 1932. *Children Who Cannot Read.* Chicago: University of Chicago Press.

Naritomi, H., Meyer, J. S., Sakai, F., Yamaguchi, F., and Shaw, T. 1979. Effects of advancing age on rCBF. *Archives of Neurology* 36:410–16.

Ojemann, G. A. 1983. Brain organization for language from the perspective of electrical stimulation mapping. *The Behavioral and Brain Sciences* 6:189–230.

Ojemann, G. A., and Whitaker, H. A. 1978. Language localization and variability. *Brain and Language* 6:239–60.

Pennington, B. F. 1986. Issues in the diagnosis and phenotype analysis of dyslexia: Implications for family studies. In *Genetics and Learning Disabilities,* ed. S. Smith. San Diego: College Hill Press, Inc.

Pennington, B. F., Lefly, D. L., Van Orden, G. C., Bookman, M. O., and Smith, S. D. 1987. Is phonology bypassed in normal or dyslexic development? *Annals of Dyslexia* 37:62–89.

Perfetti, C. A. 1985. *Reading Ability.* New York: Oxford University Press.

Prohovnik, I., Knudson, E., and Risberg, J. 1985. Theoretical evaluation and simulation test of the initial slope index for uninvasive rCBF. In *Cerebral Blood Flow & Metabolism Measurement,* eds. H. Harman and S. Hoyer. Berlin: Springer Verlag.

Rasmussen, T., and Milner, B. 1977. The role of early left-brain injury in determining lateralizations of cerebral speech functions. *Annals of the New York Academy of Sciences* 299:355–69.

Riseberg, J., Maximilian, A., and Prohovnik, I. 1977. Changes of cortical activity patterns during habituation to a reasoning task. *Neuropsychologia* 15: 793–98.

Rudel, R. G. 1985. The definition of dyslexia: Language and motor deficits. In *Dyslexia: A Neuroscientific Approach to Clinical Evaluation,* eds. F. H. Duffy and N. Geschwind. Boston/Toronto: Little, Brown and Company.

Rumsey, J. M., Dorwart, R., Vermess, M., Denckla, M. G., Kruesi, M. J. P., and Rapoport, J. L. 1986. Magnetic resonance imaging of brain anatomy in severe developmental dyslexia. *Archives on Neurology* 43:1045–1046.

Satz, P., and Van Nostrand, G. K. 1973. Developmental dyslexia: An evaluation of a theory. In *The Disabled Learner: Early Diagnosis and Intervention,* eds. P. Satz and J. Ross. Rotterdam, The Netherlands: Rotterdam University Press.

Satz, P., Taylor, H. G., Friel, J., and Fletcher, J. M. 1978. Some developmental and predictive precursors of reading disabilities: A six year follow-up. In *Dyselxia: An Appraisal of Current Knoweldge,* eds. A. L. Benton and D. Pearl. New York: Oxford University Press.

Share, D. L., McGee, R. M., Williams, S., and Silva, P. 1987. Further evidence relating to the distinction between specific reading retardation and general reading backwardness. *British Journal of Developmental Psychology* 5:35–44.

Shaywitz, S. E., Shaywitz, B. A., Fletcher, J. M., and Escobar, M. D. 1990. Prevalence of reading disability in boys and girls. *Journal of the American Medical Association* 264:998–1002.

Siegel, L. S. 1989. IQ is irrelevant to the definition of learning disabilities. *Journal of Learning Disabilities* 22(8):469–79.

Spielberger, C. D., Gorsuch, R. L., Luchene, R., Vagg, P. R., and Jacobs, G. A. 1983. *Manual for the State-Trait Anxiety Inventory (STAI)–Form Y.* Palo Alto, CA: Consulting Psychology Press.

Stanovich, K. E. 1988. Explaining the differences between the dyslexic and the garden-variety poor reader: The phonological-core variable-difference model. *Journal of Learning Disabilities* 21:590–604.

Stanovich, K. E., Cunningham, A. E., and Cramer, B. B. 1984. Assessing phonological awareness in kindergarten children: Issues of task comparability. *Journal of Experimental Child Psychology* 38:175–90.

Sur, M., Garraghty, P. E., and Roe, A. W. 1988. Experimentally induced visual projections into auditory thalamus and cortex. *Science* 242:1437–1440.

Vogel, S. 1990. Gender differences in intelligence, language, visual-motor abilities, and academic achievement in students with learning disabilities: A review of the literature. *Journal of Learning Disabilities* 23:44–52.

Wechsler, D. 1949. *Manual for the Wechsler Intelligence Scale for Children.* New York: The Psychological Corporation.

Wechsler, D. 1981. *Wechsler Adult Intelligence Scale–Revised*. New York: Psychological Corporation.

Wood, F. 1980. Theoretical, methodological, and statistical implications of the inhalation of rCBF technique for the study of brain-behavior relationships. *Brain Language* 9:1–8.

Wood, F. B. 1983. Laterality of cerebral function: Its investigation by measurement of localized brain activity. In *Cerebral Function and Asymmetry: Method, Theory and Application*, ed. J. Hellige. New York: Praeger.

Wood, F. B. 1990. Functional neuroimaging in neurobehavioral research. In *Neuromethods, Vol. 17; Neuropsychology*, eds. A. A. Boulton, G. B. Baker, and M. Hiscock. Clifton, NJ: Humana Press.

Wood, F. B., Armentrout, R., Toole, J. F., McHenry, L., and Stump, D. 1980. rCBF response during rest and memory activation in a patient with global amnesia. *Brain Language* 9:129–36.

Woodcock, R. W., and Johnson, M. B. 1977. *Woodcock–Johnson Psycho-Educational Battery*. Hingham, MA: Teaching Resources.

Chapter • 2

Neurolinguistic and Biologic Mechanisms in Dyslexia

*Bennett A. Shaywitz, Sally E. Shaywitz,
Isabelle Y. Liberman,* Jack M. Fletcher,
Donald P. Shankweiler, James S. Duncan,
Leonard Katz, Alvin M. Liberman,
David J. Francis, Lois G. Dreyer,
Stephen Crain, Susan Brady, Anne Fowler,
Leon E. Kier, Nancy S. Rosenfield,
John C. Gore, and Robert W. Makuch*

Perhaps one of the most pressing problems in learning disabilities today is in defining precisely what the entity represents. On one level this requires recognition that learning disabilities represent a heterogeneous group of disorders that must be internally differentiated from one another. Such an effort at definitional precision requires not only the elucidation of possible subgroups within learning disabilities, but also, importantly, clarifying the distinctions and interrelationships between learning disabilities (LD) and other closely related disorders, particularly, attention deficit disorder (ADD). Evidence from a number of lines of investigation now supports the belief that LD and ADD should be conceptualized as distinct entities, and though discrete, may frequently co-occur in the same child (Shaywitz and Shaywitz 1988, in press). In this report we describe the rationale, research strategy, and preliminary results from an investigation de-

Supported by grants from the National Institute of Child Health and Human Development (PO1 HD 21888 and P50 HD25802).

*Dr. Isabelle Liberman died July 19, 1990.

signed to develop a single, comprehensive classification system for the range of the most common disorders that can influence school performance, i.e., learning and attention disorders. We have taken as our primary research goal the development of a research strategy that will allow us to disentangle and elucidate the mechanisms of these two most common causes of school learning difficulties. The immediate impetus for this investigation was the recommendations of the Interagency Committee on Learning Disabilities presented in a recent Report to Congress (1987) that coincided with our own beliefs. Specifically, the Committee stated:

> A major goal of this research should be the development of a classification system that more clearly defines and diagnoses learning disabilities, conduct disorders, and attention deficit disorders, and their interrelationships. Such information is a prerequisite to the delineation of more precise and reliable strategies for treatment, remediation, and prevention that will increase the effectiveness of both research and therapy (p. 224).

We fully concur and have taken as our highest priority the development of a single reliable and valid classification system that encompasses the range of those most common, but significant, neurobehavioral disorders that interfere with school performance, including learning disabilities, attention deficit disorders, and oppositional/conduct disorder. It is our view that such a research effort focused on the clarification of definitional issues and the development of a nosology for, and elucidation of, the relationships between learning, attentional, and oppositional/conduct disorders represents the most critical need in learning disabilities research.

This report describes an investigation designed to devise and validate a classification of learning disabilities in a sample of second and third grade children. This investigation employs hypothesis-driven in-depth analytic measures of the reading process together with state-of-the-art biologic measures both to: (1) define distinct homogeneous entities and (2) gain insight into the possible mechanisms underlying reading disabilities. The development and validation of these classifications will permit the identification of those children who are specifically reading disabled and their separation from children who have other types of educational difficulties. Our investigation builds upon decades of investigations of reading disability and our research strategy should be viewed within the context of evolving concepts of dyslexia.

Evolution of the Concept of Dyslexia

What we today term dyslexia has historical roots that can be traced back to the end of the nineteenth century when the notion evolved of a specific syndrome involving the inability to read in spite of normal vision. These early reports began with the description by Kussmaul in 1877 (quoted by Hinshelwood 1896) of what he termed "word-blindness" and focused initially on reports of acquired inability to read in adults. The term *dyslexia* was first used in 1887 by Berlin (quoted by Hinshelwood 1896) but it was the Scottish ophthamologist, James Hinshelwood (1896), who differentiated complete word-blindness, alexia, from cases of partial impairment or what he termed dyslexia.

The report by Samuel T. Orton in 1925 of "Word-Blindness in School Children" heralded the modern era of our concepts of dyslexia and his report remains one of the best clinical descriptions of the disorder. Orton drew several conclusions that are still valid; he likened dyslexia to the aphasias, postulated that the problem was at the symbolic level, warned that psychometric tests unfairly penalize dyslexics, and suggested special training as a remedial step. His contention that dyslexia did not imply low intelligence and that intelligence tests do not accurately reflect the abilities of dyslexics anticipated modern definitions and make him the first advocate for dyslexic people (Orton 1925).

Orton's concepts presaged the definition of dyslexia most commonly employed today, that provided by the Research Group on Developmental Dyslexia of the World Federation of Neurology: "A disorder manifested by difficulty in learning to read despite conventional instruction, adequate intelligence, and socio-cultural opportunity. It is dependent upon fundamental cognitive disabilities which are frequently of constitutional origin" (Critchley 1970). Implicit in this definition is the exclusion of children with low intelligence or economic, cultural, or environmental disadvantage. Thus, this by now traditional concept of dyslexia has implied a distinct inherited syndrome complex not associated with preceding nervous system injury, often associated with a positive family history and not accompanied by any neurological abnormalities.

Dyslexia and Language

The symptom complex denoted by the term *dyslexia* focuses on difficulties with language and words—their use, significance, meaning, pronunciation, and spelling—and the problems generated by this lexical difficulty. Good evidence from a number of lines of investigation indicates that the prime modality affected in dyslexia is that of language. The intimate connection of the reading process to language has been demonstrated repeatedly. Poor readers have an increased incidence of delayed speech (Frith 1981), a finding that characterized as many as 15% of the poor readers in the Isle of Wight studies (Rutter, Tizard, and Whitmore 1970). Disabled readers experience difficulties in labelling or naming common objects; they are dysnomic (Katz 1982; Denckla and Rudel 1976; Wolf 1981). Poor readers, particularly, have difficulty appreciating that words are composed of smaller units in the form of syllables, morphemes, and especially phonemes (Liberman 1971; Liberman et al. 1974). The work of Vellutino, and Liberman (1979), and her associates has provided data to support a language-based theory of reading disability that focuses on the phonological component of language (Liberman et al. 1982; Mann and Liberman 1984; Shankweiler et al. 1979; Vellutino 1979).

Such evidence leads us to certain working assumptions about language and reading:

1. Language communicates meanings mediated by phonological and syntactic structures. Language is thus set apart from communicative systems of other kinds, as for example, those that use pictures.

2. An orthography represents language. The point here is that writing is based on language; it is not a wholly different communication system.

3. Alphabetic forms of writing (which are our concern here) represent the phonology of the language. An alphabetic orthography transcribes the language in ways that correspond to certain of its natural "seams," with the consonants and vowels supplying the basic building blocks for words.

4. Reading is harder to acquire than speech. If reading were as natural as speaking, everyone who speaks the language would also be able to read and write. Clearly, this does not happen; reading always follows speech production and comprehension and often takes several years to master. The fact that difficulties in apprehension of spoken language are not readily discerned in reading-disabled individuals indicates that reading must, in some way, place greater stress on the cognitive-linguistic system.

Our research strategy is guided by the hypothesis that language processes and abilities are distinct from other cognitive processes. The language apparatus forms a biologically coherent system—in Fodor's terms, a "module" (Fodor 1983)—that is distinguished from other portions of the cognitive apparatus by special brain structures and by other anatomical specializations (Liberman and Mattingly 1989; Milner 1975; Studdert-Kennedy and Shankweiler 1970). An extension of the hypothesis supposes that the language faculty is itself composed of several autonomous subsystems: the phonology, the syntax, and the semantic system together with the processors that serve them, the working memory, and the parser. The concept of language as a hierarchical system of components has important implications for understanding how reading is acquired and for interpreting the difficulties that arise in poor readers. A modular view of the language apparatus raises the possibility that any number of components of language processing may be the source of reading disorder (Crain and Shankweiler 1988; Mann 1986; Mann, Liberman, and Shankweiler 1980; Liberman, Shankweiler, and Liberman 1989). On the other hand, the fact that these components are related in a hierarchical fashion allows that a complex of symptoms of reading disorder may derive from a single affected component.

Issues Addressed

In addition to the overriding classification problems, this study addresses several specific issues concerning cognitive and biological mechanisms in reading disability.

1. Is all reading disability specific to the linguistic system? Broadly speaking, there are three ways in which reading and language might be related. It is possible that: (a) all types of reading disorder are in the language domain; (b) only some types are; or (c) none are. Since we do not know which of these possibilities is correct, it is essential that assessment procedures be designed to distinguish subtypes of reading disorder where these exist, and to find out as much as possible about the mechanisms of reading within these subtypes. Thus the neurolinguistic and neuropsychological testing must include not only language measures but also parallel nonlanguage tests that yield, in so far as possible, pure measures of other cognitive abilities, so that language and nonlanguage abilities are not confounded with one another.

2. If not all reading disabilities are linguistically based, what characterizes those that have other sources? Are there different genetic-neurologic profiles for the different types of reading disability? It is possible that there are different subtypes of reading disability that differ from one another in the affected component. (a) Is there, for example, a specific phonologic type of reading disorder?—Problems that many poor readers have in abstracting and manipulating phonological segments of words might suggest that there is; (b) Is there a specific syntactic type?—Poor readers' problems in interpreting complex sentences in spoken language raises this question; (c) Is there a specific semantic type?—Poor readers' difficulties in finding names of objects can be a manifestation of a semantic deficit.

3. Alternatively, a general language deficit may stem from a deficit in language processing capacity rather than a deficit in structural knowledge at a particular level of language. The root cause can lie in a low-level component yet can give rise to manifestations that spread up-

ward throughout the system (Liberman and Shankweiler 1985; Shankweiler and Crain 1986). Thus, the problem can be linguistic, but can implicate disordered processes subsidiary to language rather than missing or malformed language structures, per se. Specifically, we might expect to find disturbances affecting the working memory system, the attentional system, or the metacognitive system.

4. Finally, we test for the possibility that apparent language problems may stem from a general processing deficit cutting across different cognitive domains. Our tests will allow us to determine whether there are underlying deficits in attention, memory, perception, or metacognition.

Classification of Dyslexia

Why devote this energy to developing a nosology or classification system for reading disabilities? A basic assumption in our proposed classification research is that there are children who show similarities and/or differences in their neurobehavioral abilities/disabilities. By identifying these similarities and/or differences, in these "types" of children, we believe that a better understanding of etiologies, prognoses, and treatments will be provided, represented in part by the issues outlined in the previous section. However, the issues can only be addressed adequately in the context of a classification of learning and reading disability in children.

Classification systems are the fundamental first step in any scientific enterprise (see Morris and Fletcher 1988). Their importance is exemplified by this quotation from Stephen Jay Gould's book, *Wonderful Life* (1989):

> Taxonomy is a fundamental and dynamic science dedicated to exploring the causes of relationships and similarities among organisms. Classifications are theories about the basis of natural order, not dull catalogues compiled only to avoid chaos (p. 98).

Gleick (1989), reviewing Gould's book, further emphasized the importance of classification systems:

> . . . the work of placing . . . in categories, carefully weighing similarities and differences and occasionally discarding an old category and inventing a new one leads, inexorably, to a new view . . . (p. 41).

A classification system addressing the interrelationship of learning, reading, and other childhood disabilities is the critical first step if we are to examine neurobiological mechanisms of the various possible subtypes of reading disability (if any) and develop a rational management for each potential subtype.

In our investigation, the development of a nosology is informed by hypothesis-driven models of language and attention. While we recognize that there are other possible components or models for learning disabilities and attention disorders, we have selected components of language and attention as the two major models supported in research studies to date. Formation of the classifications of learning and attention disorders derives from Skinner's framework for classification research (Skinner 1981; Fletcher, Morris, and Francis in press). A key tenet is that any classification represents basically a scientific theory that then must be subjected to empirical testing for validation. This framework includes three different components, each of which underlies an integrated paradigm for classification research.

First, Skinner describes the theory formulation component. This component involves decisions concerning the kinds of variables that are used for a classification and the specific groups that are hypothesized to exist. In this component the investigators propose a priori groups that are hypothesized to exist as well as proposing structural models that provide linkages among these proposed groups or hypothesized subtypes. It is at this stage of the classification process that classification attributes are selected and their relationship to external variables hypothesized. It should be noted that in the Skinner model, hypothesized types are ideal representations presumed to exist in the population. Types are generated in part to establish modal expectations, but also to establish relationships with other classes of the phenomena of interest. This process leads directly to a sampling strategy and selection of major attributes representing how types are presumably similar and different. Secondly, the internal validation component represents the assessment of reliability (consistency of diagnosis), coverage (applicability of diagnosis for all children), and homogeneity (similarity of group members to one another). This component employs several different methods including: split samples and the use of additional attributes; multiple clustering comparisons; and the use of Monte Carlo tests (Morris, Satz, and Blashfield 1981). Third, the external validity component involves the evaluation of a reliable classification system against external criteria, which addresses whether the groups differ from one another according to biological markers, response to treatment, or other indices used to study these groups.

METHODS

Sampling Strategy

No consensus exists concerning the most appropriate criteria for identifying disabled readers. Some definitions favor the use of discrepancy formulas, while others simply establish the presence of "average" IQ and "deficient" achievement regardless of the discrepancy of IQ and achievement. At this point, empirical studies show few, if any, differences between disabled readers who meet or do not meet discrepancy-based criteria (Rutter 1978; Taylor, Satz, and Friel 1979). Consequently, in order to develop a classification that will identify severely disabled readers, it is necessary to sample according to both types of definitions. Moreover, since many reading-disabled children also have problems in mathematics, it is necessary to obtain reading-disabled children with and without mathematics disabilities. The use of mathematically disabled children who vary in reading ability also adds an important contrast group, particularly since empirical studies consistently show differences among learning-disabled children according to patterns of word recognition and computational skills (Fletcher 1985; Rourke 1985). Since many reading-disabled children also have attentional deficits, we have not based our inclusion/exclusion criteria on attentional skills. However, we are recruiting a contrast group of attentionally impaired children without concomitant achievement problems to help evaluate the influence of attentional impairment on reading disabilities.

Therefore, criteria for sample selection include groups of children meeting criteria for disability based on:

A. Alternative definitions of disability including:
   1. discrepancy between ability and achievement
   2. low achievement irrespective of a discrepancy
B. Achievement area affected
   1. reading alone
   2. mathematics alone
   3. reading and mathematics both affected
C. Attentional deficit without an accompanying academic deficit.

A total of six groups of children are selected utilizing a combination of definitional and achievement criteria—three groups of disabled children on the basis of an IQ–achievement discrepancy and three groups of children on the basis of low achievement in the three academic areas indicated above. A seventh group is selected on the basis of an attentional deficit without an accompanying academic deficit. This group is divided equally between children who meet criteria for ADD with hyperactivity (ADDH) and ADD without hyperactivity (ADDNoH).

Our sampling strategy also includes a group of average children who do not fulfill any of the criteria for academic or attentional disability and a group of below average/mentally deficient children. Therefore, for classification purposes, nine a priori groups are included in the sample:

1. Discrepancy (ability/achievement) in reading
2. Discrepancy (ability/achievement) in mathematics
3. Discrepancy (ability/achievement) in reading and mathematics
4. Low achievement (irrespective of a discrepancy) in reading
5. Low achievement (irrespective of a discrepancy) in mathematics
6. Low achievement (irrespective of a discrepancy) in reading and mathematics
7. Attention deficit disorder without accompanying achievement deficit
8. Average (do not meet criteria for groups 1–7)
9. Mentally deficient/below average with IQ in 60–79 range.

The addition of groups 8 and 9 addresses two important areas necessary to be considered in the development of a classification system. These are: (1) the ability of the classification system to differentiate disabled from non-disabled children and (2) whether children who are reading disabled and have an IQ in the below average range can be differentiated from children who are reading disabled and have average ability. A contrast group of "average" non-disabled children is needed to ensure that any comparisons will differentiate impaired from unimpaired children. Since some of the behavioral and biological measures lack age-norms, this group also is important for internal and external validity studies.

In order to address the second issue, another contrast group, a below average/mentally deficient group is also essential to the development of a classification system. The definition of this group deserves comment. Traditionally, such a contrast group has been defined as mentally retarded (MR) children who do not meet inclusion criteria for the learning disability samples. Such a group requires an IQ score of 70 or below, developmental onset, and adaptive behavior consistent with this level of functioning. The use of a similarly defined MR sample in the current project created a methodological gap because some children with IQs between 70 and 80 would be eliminated.

The problem is that IQ criteria for defining "average" or "mentally deficient" are arbitrary and often do not correspond closely with other equally relevant criteria. Average can be defined in many ways: (1) an IQ above 90 on the WISC–R was defined as "average" by Wechsler, (2) an IQ above 85, i.e., one standard deviation below the population mean, is used by many researchers; and (3) an IQ above 70 represents children not considered mentally retarded. Again, such a criterion is arbitrary. To be adequate as a contrast group in this project, children included should be representative of the distribution of subjects falling directly below the operational definition of "average" to ensure adequate representation of such subjects. Therefore, the classification question, for example, is to differentiate a reading-disabled child who has an IQ of 80 from a below-average child with an IQ under 80. This question is important for classification of the groups of children under investigation, since children with a "specific" developmental disability have traditionally been differentiated from those children with a "general" disability. The question at issue is whether an IQ score of 80 represents a natural break between such groups. The selection of this contrast sample will provide data for the empirical analysis of these questions.

In summary the sampling strategy we followed casts a wide net to assure that the groups are inclusive enough so that the various possible subtypes may emerge. In addition, the sampling strategy allows us to address important questions concerning:

1. distinctions between discrepancy based and low achieving groups of reading-disabled children
2. distinctions between reading disability in isolation and in combination with other achievement deficiencies
3. the influence of attentional deficits
4. the empirical validity of the traditional practice of excluding individuals with below 80 IQ.

Finally, our sampling strategy will ensure that the classification system that emerges will differentiate disabled from non-disabled children.

Test Batteries

Four test batteries have been developed for use in this study. The first, the screening battery, is used to select the subjects according to selection criteria described in the preceding sections. It is composed of the Wechsler Intelligence Scale for Children–Revised (WISC–R, Wechsler 1974), the Reading, Arithmetic, and Spelling subtests of the Wide Range Achievement Test (WRAT, Jastak and Jastak 1978), the Reading, Mathematics, and Written Language subtests of the Woodcock–Johnson Psycho-Educational Battery (W–J, Woodcock and Johnson 1977), pure tone audiometric screening, and a test of visual acuity.

The second test battery contains the measures used for reading and spelling assessment. Reading assessment includes two sections, one relating to decoding skills and the other to contextual reading and comprehension. Decoding skills are tested by means of the Letter Word Identification subtest of the W–J, the word recognition subtest of the WRAT, and the phonic patterns subtest of the Decoding Skills Test (DST, Richardson and DiBenedetto 1985). Contextual reading and comprehension is assessed with the comprehension subtest of the W–J, the revised Gray Oral Reading Test (GORT–R, Wiederholt and

Bryant 1986) and the Formal Reading Inventory (FRI, Wiederholt 1986). The FRI provides standardized norms for silent reading comprehension, using the very stories and questions making up Form B of the GORT–R. The FRI has the additional advantage of providing two parallel forms (C and D), each with stories and comprehension questions increasing in difficulty from 1 to 13 years. We have recorded Form C on audio tape for oral presentation to test listening comprehension. Thus we have one parallel set of stories to test oral reading fluency, oral reading comprehension, silent reading comprehension, and listening comprehension. Spelling achievement will be assessed by means of the Spelling subtest of the WRAT and by the Larsen–Hammill Test of Written Spelling (TWS, Larsen and Hammill 1976).

The third test battery, the Neurolinguistic and Neuropsychological Battery, provides the core of the basic research tests of language and cognitive function, which will supply much of the data for the classification development. It includes eight sections, each with multiple subsections, reflecting the major dimensions of the reading task. These include phonological awareness, short-term memory, vocabulary and word-finding, speech perception, speech production, morphological awareness, syntactic comprehension, and attention.

The fourth battery, the Behavior and Environmental Information Battery, is represented by a series of instruments that provide critical background information about each child. This battery includes information provided by the child's parent(s): the Yale Children's Inventory (YCI, Shaywitz et al. 1986; Shaywitz et al. 1988), the Child Behavior Checklist (CBCL, Achenbach and Edelbrock l984), the Henderson Environmental Learning Process Scale (HELPS, Henderson, Bergan and Hurt 1972; Valencia, Henderson and Rankin 1985), the Diagnostic Interview Schedule for Children, revised (DISC, Costello et al. 1984); the child's classroom teacher: the Multigrade Inventory for Teachers (MIT, Shaywitz 1986), the End of Year Evaluation (EYE, Shaywitz 1986), the Conners Teacher Questionnaire (ATQ, Goyette, Conners, and Ulrich 1978); and by the children themselves: the Neuromaturational Assessment Scales (NMAS, Shaywitz et al. 1984), the Edinburgh Handedness Inventory (Oldfield 1971), and Harter's Perceived Self-Competence Scales (Harter 1982).

RESULTS

Complete data are available on the first 71 children entered into the study at the time of this presentation and the interpretation of the findings must be viewed very cautiously. We first analyzed the correlations between a number of the reading measures and those in the neurolinguistic test battery on all 71 children (see table I). Scores on the Decoding Skills Test, a measure of mastery of the alphabetic principle, are related significantly to the child's ability to perform on the word attack test of the Woodcock–Johnson, his or her ability to read orally and silently (as measured by the GORT–R and the FRI), and the child's ability to discriminate the morphological components of words. However, at the ages assessed, the child's vocabulary, as measured on the Peabody Picture Vocabulary Test, did not appear to be related to orthographic ability or overall measures of reading.

We next analyzed the 71 children according to whether they satisfied criteria for reading disability, defined by either a discrepancy criterion or low achievement. Children in the reading disabled (RD, $n = 23$) group were similar in ability to those in the non-reading disabled (No RD, $n = 42$) group (see figure 1). Scale scores on the Yale Children's Inventory indicated that the mothers of the RD group viewed their offspring as more inattentive, more impulsive, and exhibiting more academic and language problems than did the mothers of the No RD children (see figure 2). These findings are not surprising since many of the children in the RD group were also diagnosed as having attention deficit disorder (ADD). It is interesting that activity levels did not differ, suggesting that many of these children with RD and ADD can be categorized as having ADD without hyperactivity (Lahey and Carlson in press).

Results on the reading and neurolinguistic test battery can be classified broadly within four general patterns representing the degree of difference between the RD and No RD groups. In Pattern #1 (see figure

Table I. Correlations Between Neurolinguistic and Reading Measures

Decoding Skills Test X	*Gray Oral Reading Test X*
WJ14 .74	FRI .82
MOR .72	MOR .75
GORT .70	DST .73
FRI .69	WJ14 .73
Morphologic Awareness X	*PPVT X*
GORT .75	No significant correlations
DST .72	
FRI .66	
WJ14 .64	

Correlations are Pearson r
WJ14—Woodcock Johnson word attack
MOR—morphological awareness
GORT—Gray Oral Reading Test–Revised
FRI—Formal Reading Inventory
DST—Decoding Skills Test
PPVT—Peabody Picture Vocabulary Test

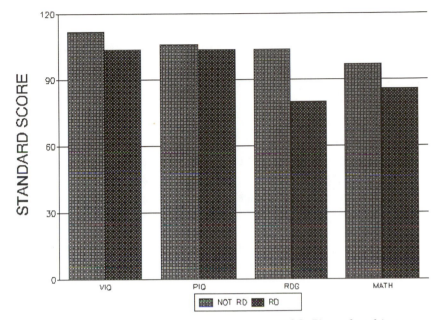

Figure 1. Verbal and peformance ability (WISC–R) and achievement (Woodcock–Johnson Reading and Math Cluster scores) in reading disabled (RD) compared to children without reading disability. Reading disability diagnosed on the basis of either a discrepancy criteria or low achievement or both.

3a), exemplified by tests that are believed to tap phonologic awareness (Decoding Skills Test, Auditory Analysis Test [AAT], Rosner and Simon 1971), RD childrens' scores are 30–40% of those of No RD children. Differences between RD and No RD are not quite as marked in Pattern #2 (see figure 3b), exemplified by scores on the GORT–R and FRI, and are even less pronounced in Pattern #3 (see figure 3c), illustrated by tests of morphological awareness and verbal short-term memory. No differences are observed between RD and No RD on tests of vocabulary (PPVT) or visual motor integration, designated as Pattern #4 (see figure 3d).

We then analyzed the cohort with the view toward separating reading disabled into those who satisfied discrepancy criteria only (Dis) and those who were classified as reading disabled not only because of discrepancy but because of low achievement (Dis/LA) as well. Figure 4 indicates the performance of all three groups (No RD, Dis, Dis/LA) on representative measures from the reading and neurolinguistic battery. Reading-disabled children, whether Dis alone or Dis/LA performed worse than No RD children on phonologic measures (DST and AAT) and oral reading (GORT–R). Within these measures, children with Dis/LA performed worse than those reading-disabled children di-

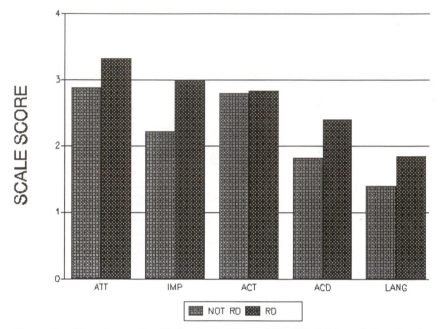

Figure 2.   Parent reports of behavior in RD and No RD children defined as in figure 1. Scores are scale scores on the Yale Children's Inventory.

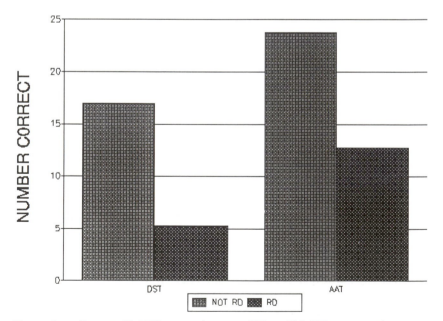

Figure 3a.   Pattern #1: Differences between RD and No RD on tests of tapping phonologic awareness: Decoding Skills Test and the Auditory Analysis Test.

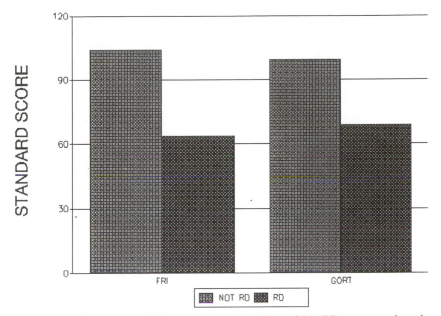

Figure 3b.   Pattern #2: Differences between RD and No RD on tests of reading: Gray Oral Reading Test and Formal Reading Inventory.

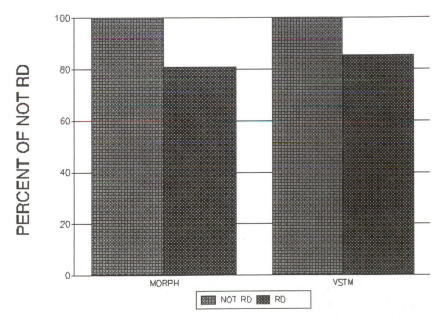

Figure 3c.   Pattern #3: Differences between RD and No RD on tests of morphological awareness and verbal short-term memory.

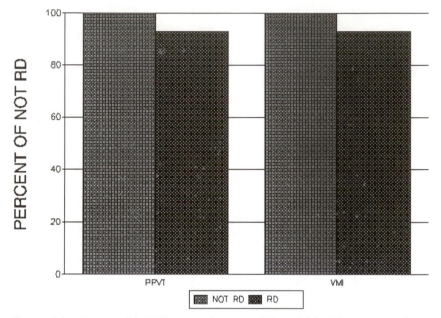

Figure 3d. Pattern #4: Differences between RD and No RD on tests of vocabulary (Peabody Picture Vocabulary Test) and visual motor integration (Beery Test of Visual Motor Integration).

agnosed based only on discrepancy criteria. On a measure of verbal short-term memory, those in the Dis group were similar to these in No RD though Dis/LA children performed less well than both. These findings suggest that those children designated as RD on the basis of discrepancy criteria perform better than those satisfying criteria for both discrepancy and low achievement in reading. However, such findings may simply reflect lower ability in the Dis/LA group. Thus, scores on ability (WISC–R) and achievement (Woodcock–Johnson) measures are shown for the three groups (No RD, Dis, Dis/LA) in figure 5; children in the Dis/LA group performed the poorest on all these measures.

DISCUSSION

In this report we have focused on the rationale and research strategy of a classification system for learning disabilities, proposing a dual level, hierarchical model as shown in figure 6. At Level I children are classified into major forms of learning disability according to areas of academic impairment. Three major subgroups of learning disabilities are considered: disorders of reading, mathematics, and both reading and mathematics. It is recognized that children can have problems in spell-

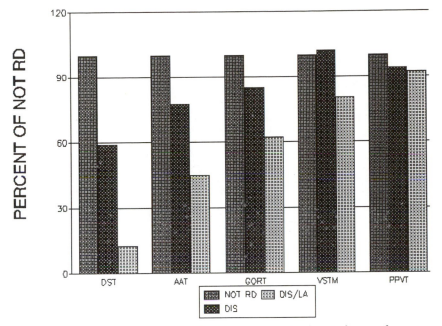

Figure 4. Performance on representative tests from the reading and neurolinguistic test battery. Three groups are considered: children without reading disability (No RD); reading disability diagnosed using discrepancy criteria alone (Dis); and reading disability diagnosed using both discrepancy and low achievement critieria (Dis/LA). Reading-disabled children perform less well than No RD on measures tapping phonologic awareness (Decoding Skills Test, DST; Auditory Analysis Test, AAT) and reading (Gray Oral Reading Test, GORT). Dis/LA perform the worst on these measures and verbal short-term memory (STM). No differences are observed on a measure of vocabulary (Peabody Picture Vocabulary Test, PPV).

ing, writing, and other areas, either in conjunction with or in isolation from these disorders. However, these three groups of children encompass the majority of those with learning disabilities. Since children with learning disorders also have problems with attention, a comparison group of ADD children (without reading or mathematics disability) is included. Two other comparison groups of "normal" and below average/mentally deficient children are included to control for decisions about IQ and achievement criteria. At Level I the objective is to differentiate subgroups at the level of major disability: reading, mathematics, attention, low IQ, no disability. At Level II children with reading disability are classified into subtypes based on their performance on an analytic test battery of neurolinguistic measures designed to probe the language module. Hypothesized subtypes of reading include phonology, phonology/short term memory, and general cognitive. These hy-

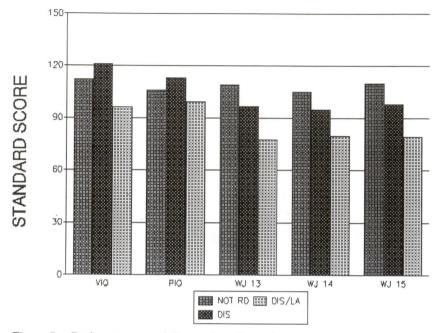

Figure 5. Performance on ability and reading achievement measures. Groups defined as in figure 4. Dis/LA consistently perform worse than Dis alone and No RD in verbal and performance IQ (VIQ, PIQ of WISC–R) and in reading subtests of the Woodcock–Johnson.

pothesized subtypes can then be further validated using neurobiological measures including quantitative neuroimaging techniques and electrophysiological measures.

The thrust of the classification is always to proceed from the general to the more specific. Thus, as we proceed from Level I to Level II, our classification system becomes increasingly more precise and fine-grained. We begin by considering the broad cognitive grouping "learning disability," but then, within this grouping, focus on reading disability alone, and as a final step delineate the subtypes within reading disability. Consequently, our study not only addresses possible reading subtypes, but also provides a potential validation of the construct of learning disability.

The data reported here are those available on the first 71 children to enter the study; our results are therefore preliminary and, as noted earlier, must be viewed cautiously. Our findings indicate that, compared to children who have no reading disability, children diagnosed as reading disabled, either on the basis of an ability-achievement discrepancy or because of low achievement, perform significantly less well on tests tapping phonologic awareness, reading comprehension, and

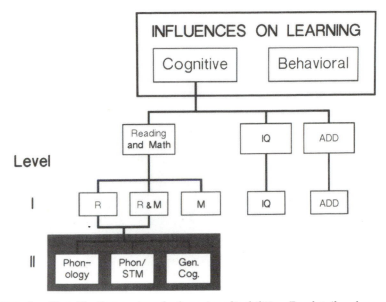

Figure 6.   Classification system for learning disabilities. For details, please see text.

verbal short-term memory. They perform comparably to non-reading disabled children on measures of vocabulary and visual motor integration. RD children appear to exhibit their poorest performance on those tests that tap mastery of the alphabetic principle, such as the Decoding Skills Test or tests of phonologic awareness, such as the Auditory Analysis Test. Thus, even at this early stage of our investigation, the data appear to support the belief that reading disability is related to disturbances in the phonologic component of the language module.

At the outset we indicated that current evidence suggests that both learning disabilities and attention deficit disorder can be conceptualized as distinct diagnostic entities that may frequently co-occur in the same child. A primary need exists (a) to better understand each of these disorders including specifically their etiology, pathogenesis, course, and response to treatment; and (b) to clarify the distinctions and interrelationships between learning disabilities and other closely related disorders, specifically attention deficit disorder. Reflecting this need, in more recent investigations we have broadened the scope of our classification enterprise to incorporate children with attentional and oppositional/conduct disorders. These newer studies focus on developing a classification system for children with attention and oppositional/conduct disorders, both with and without learning disabilities. For attention deficit disorder we have proposed the dual level hierarchical model outlined in figure 7. At Level I we have identified major

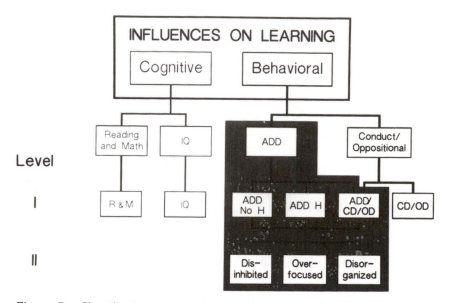

Figure 7. Classification system for attention deficit disorder. For details, please see text.

groups of ADD children with and without hyperactivity who may or may not have co-occurring disorders of learning (reading, mathematics, mental deficiency) and behavior (oppositional/conduct disorder). At Level II we have subdivided the ADD children into three postulated cognitive types (disinhibited, overfocused, disorganized) based on laboratory assessments of attention suggested by Cooley and Morris (in press). At Level I our study is designed to disentangle attention disorder from oppositional/conduct disorder and then at Level II to proceed to elucidate the subtypes within attention deficit disorder. As in the dyslexia investigation, we will validate this typology using biologic measures.

Overall, a unified approach is utilized for the learning disability and attentional studies. Parallel strategies and approaches are employed relating to subject selection, determination of a priori study groups, selection of measures, selection of procedures and statistical analysis; as far as possible the same measures are administered to the children in both these newer studies and our ongoing dyslexia project. This strategy of common procedures and measures significantly increases the power of our ability to develop a single comprehensive classification system for learning and attention disorders. Incorporation of behavioral, cognitive, and biologic measures in both classification enterprises should permit the emerging subtypes to be characterized in meaningful ways.

IMPLICATIONS

For at least two decades, members of our investigative group have been seriously concerned with learning and attention problems in children. It has become increasingly evident that both reading disability and attention deficit disorder each represent a heterogeneous group of disorders. Significant advances in our understanding of the basic mechanisms and in determining the most effective therapy depend upon the delineation of homogeneous subtypes of each of these groups of disorders. In this report we have outlined how our investigative group has conceptualized this process. We have provided a detailed overview of the rationale and study design for a classification of reading disability and indicated how a parallel classification system is being developed for attention deficit disorder.

A major research issue is the relationship between reading disability and attention deficit disorder. While it is clear that these disorders co-occur in many children, the nature of this relationship is still very much an open research question. We realized that it would be much more meaningful to develop a classification system that would be applicable to both reading disability and attention deficit disorder. A primary concern was the need to maintain the integrity of the hypothesized models for each of these disorders and yet to develop a classification system that would be relevant to both groups of disorders. Our approach to this problem was to employ measures reflecting current hypotheses about reading disability and attention deficit disorder. In each component of the classification study each subject receives all the measures developed for that arm of the classification; for example, all children in the reading study receive all the linguistic measures. However, there are also numerous bridges between the studies built into the research design so that, for example, children in the reading study also are examined using a subset of the measures used in the attention disorder classification. Similarly, children in the attention disorder study will be assessed using a subset of the linguistic test battery. Not only do the studies share measures, but a common classification framework serves to bind the reading and attention disorder classifications.

Our research enterprise, encompassing the spectrum of learning and attention disorders that influence school performance, is summarized in figure 8. Each study utilizes distinct and separate populations. In the study of learning disabilities the sample includes children with a variety of learning and attention problems. However, the focus is on reading problems. Analytic and biologic measures are employed to be able to better delineate and differentiate the subtypes of reading disability. In the companion study of attention disorder, a separate and large population of children with attention disorder and related learn-

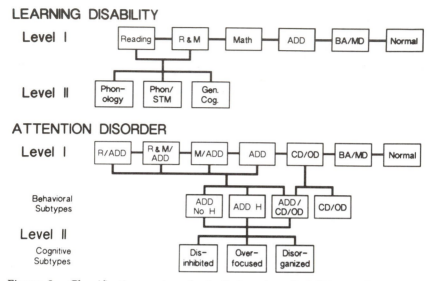

Figure 8. Classification system for both learning disabilities and attention deficit disorder. For details, please see text.

ing and behavioral disorders are recruited and assessed. However, in this case the emphasis is on attention disorder and analytic measures of attention are utilized to develop, at Level II, a typology of attention disorder.

The generalizability of both the studies of learning and attention can be addressed utilizing data from the Connecticut Longitudinal study. This epidemiological and longitudinal study adds further depth and cohesiveness to our classification studies by providing an estimate of the prevalence and stability of the types of learning disabilities and attention disorder. Longitudinal assessment of our epidemiological sample will provide information on the ontogeny of patterns of ability, achievement, and of different types of learning disability and attention disorder in an unselected sample of school children.

Figures 9 and 10 summarize how we have conceptualized the process of proceeding from the global problem of school learning difficulties to the development of a reliable and valid classification system that encompasses both reading disability and attention deficit disorder. We begin with the global problem of school learning difficulties (see figure 9). We hypothesize that there are three major influences on learning—cognitive, attentional and behavioral. At a still finer level, the cognitive influences are represented by reading, mathematics, and other disabilities. The attentional influences are further subdivided into ADD with and without hyperactivity subgroups, while the behavioral influences are represented by oppositional/conduct disorders. At each

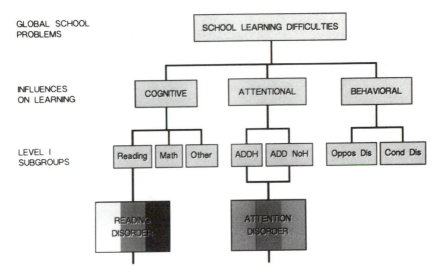

Figure 9. Overall view of classification enterprise. For details, please see text.

step, the process becomes increasingly more precise so that for example, once reading disability (or attention deficit disorder) is differentiated from other disabilities, we focus on reading disability and attention disorder for further analytic studies. We then can determine specific subtypes that compose reading disability and attention disorder.

We have hypothesized three subtypes of reading disability and three subtypes of attention disorder (see figure 10). Once we have de-

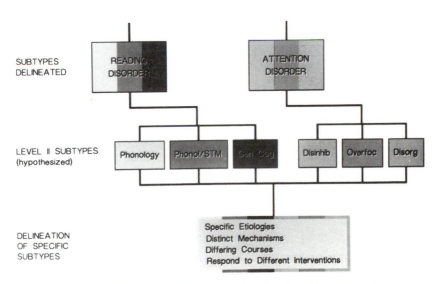

Figure 10. Overall view of classification. For details, please see text.

lineated, defined, and validated each of the specific subtypes, then and only then can we proceed to consider the specific etiologies, distinct mechanisms, and what are likely to be different interventions for each of the specific subtypes of reading and attention disorder.

Together, both arms of the classification, that for reading disability and that for ADD, will link to form the broad and solid foundation necessary for the development of a comprehensive classification system for these disorders. Such a strategy also offers the potential to provide insights into the nature of the relationship between linguistic and attentional function, both in reading and in attention deficit disorder. We believe that the end result will be the development of a nosology that is not limited to either reading or attention disorder but incorporates both of these entities. Delineation of more homogeneous subtypes represents a significant step in the development of rational and effective intervention strategies for the broad range of learning and attention disorders.

REFERENCES

Achenbach, T. M., and Edelbrock, C. S. 1984. *Manual for the Child Behavior Checklist and Revised Child Behavior Profile.* Burlington, VT.

Cooley, E. L., and Morris, R. in press. Attention in children: A neuropsychologically-based model of assessment. *Developmental Neuropsychology.*

Costello, A., Edelbrock, C., Dulcan, M., and Kalas, R. 1984. *Testing of the NIMH Diagnostic Interview Schedule for Children (DISC in a Clinical Population: Final Report.)* National Institute of Mental Health.

Crain, S., and Shankweiler, D. 1988. Syntactic complexity and reading acquisition. In *Linguistic Complexity and Text Comprehension,* eds. A. Davison and G. M. Green. New Jersey: Lawrence Erlbaum Assoc.

Critchley, M. 1970. *The Dyslexic Child.* Springfield, IL: Charles C Thomas.

Denckla, M. B., and Rudel, R. G. 1976. Naming of object drawings by dyslexic and other learning disabled children. *Brain and Language* 3:1–16.

Fletcher, J. M. 1985. External validation of learning disability subtypes. In *Neuropsychology of Learning Disabilities: Essentials of Subtypal Analysis,* ed. B. P. Rourke. New York: Guilford.

Fletcher, J. M., Morris, R. D., and Francis, D. J. in press. Methodological issues in the classification of attention and related disorders. *Journal of Learning Disabilities.*

Fodor, J. A. 1983. *The Modularity of Mind.* Cambridge: MIT Press.

Frith, U. 1981. Experimental approaches to developmental dyslexia. *Psychological Research* 43:97–109.

Gleick, J. 1989. Reviewing Stephan Jay Gould's "Wonderful Life." October 22, 1989. *The New York Times.* (Book Review).

Gould, S. J. 1989. *Wonderful Life: The Burgess Shale and the Nature of History.* New York: Norton.

Goyette, C. H., Conners, C. K., and Ulrich, R. F. 1978. Normative data on revised Conners teacher and parent rating scales. *Journal of Abnormal Child Psychology* 6:221–36.

Harter, S. 1982. The perceived competence scale for children. *Child Development* 53:87–97.

Henderson, R. W., Bergan, J. R., and Hurt, M., Jr. 1972. The development and validation of the Henderson environmental learning process scale. *Journal of Social Psychology* 88:185–96.

Hinshelwood, J. 1896. A case of dyslexia: A peculiar form of word-blindness. *The Lancet*, 1451–1454.

Interagency Committee on Learning Disabilities. 1987. *Learning Disabilities: A Report to the U.S. Congress.* Washington, D.C.: U.S. Government Printing Office.

Jastak, J., and Jastak, S. 1978. The wide range achievement test 1978. In *Manual of Instructions*, revised ed. Wilmington: Jastak Associates.

Katz, R. B. 1982. Phonological deficiencies in children with reading disability: Evidence from an object-naming task. Unpublished doctoral dissertation, University of Connecticut: Storrs, CT.

Lahey, B. B., and Carlson, K. in press. Validity of a diagnostic category of attention deficit disorder without hyperactivity: A review of the literature. *Journal of Learning Disabilities.*

Larsen, S., and Hammill, D. 1976. *Test of Written Spelling.* Austin, TX: Pro-Ed.

Liberman, A. M., and Mattingly, I. G. 1989. A specialization for speech perception. *Science* 243:489–94.

Liberman, I. Y. 1971. Basic research in speech and lateralization of language: Some implications for reading disability. *Bulletin of the Orton Society* 21:71–87.

Liberman, I. Y., Mann, V. A., Shankweiler, D., and Werfelman, M. 1982. Children's memory for recurring linguistic and non-linguistic material in relation to reading ability. *Cortex* 18:367–75.

Liberman, I. Y., Shankweiler, D., Fischer, F. W., and Carter, B. 1974. Explicit syllable and phoneme segmentation in the young child. *Experimental Child Psychology* 18:201–12.

Mann, V. A. 1986. Why some children encounter reading problems: The contribution of difficulties with language processing and language sophistication to early reading disability. In *Educational Perspectives on Learning Disabilities,* eds. J. K. Torgesen and B. Y. Wong. New York: Academic Press.

Mann, V. A., and Liberman, I. Y. 1984. Phonological awareness and verbal short-term memory. *Journal of Learning Disabilities* 10:592–99.

Mann, V. A., Liberman, I. Y., and Shankweiler, D. 1980. Children's memory for sentences and word strings in relation to reading ability. *Memory and Cognition* 8:329–35.

Milner, B. 1975. Hemispheric specialization: Scopes and limits. In *The Neurosciences Third Study Program,* eds. F. O. Schmitt and F. G. Worden. Cambridge: MIT Press.

Morris, R. D., and Fletcher, J. M. 1988. Classification in neuropsychology: A theoretical framework and research paradigm. *Journal of Clinical and Experimental Neuropsychology* 10:640–58.

Morris, R. D., Satz, P., and Blashfield, R. 1981. Neuropsychology and cluster analysis: Problems and pitfalls. *Journal of Clinical and Experimental Neuropsychology* 3:79–99.

Oldfield, R. C. 1971. The assessment of handedness: The Edinburgh Inventory. *Neuropsychologia* 9:97–113.

Orton, S. T. 1925. "Word-blindness" in school children. *Archives of Neurology and Psychiatry* 14:581–615.

Richardson, E., and DiBenedetto, B. 1985. *Decoding Skills Test.* Parkton, MD: York Press.

Rosner, J., and Simon, D. 1971. The auditory analysis test: An initial report. *Journal of Learning Disabilities* 4:384–92.

Rourke, B. P. 1989. *Nonverbal Learning Disabilities: The Syndrome and the Model.* New York: Guilford.

Rutter, M. 1978. Prevalence and types of dyslexia. In *Dyslexia, An Appraisal of Current Knowledge* eds. A. L. Benton and D. Pearl. New York: Oxford University Press.

Rutter, M., Tizard, J., and Whitmore, K. 1970. *Education, Health, and Behavior.* London: Longman.

Shankweiler, D., and Crain, S. 1986. Language mechanisms and reading disorders: A modular approach. *Cognition* 24:136–68.

Shankweiler, D., Liberman, I. Y., Mann, V. A., Fowler, A., and Fisher, F. W. 1979. The speech code and learning to read: Human learning and memory. *Journal of Experimental Psychology* 5:531–45.

Shaywitz, S. E. 1986. Early recognition of vulnerability–EREV. Technical report to Connecticut State Department of Education.

Shaywitz, S. E., and Shaywitz, B. A. 1988. Attention deficit disorder: Current perspectives. *Learning Disabilities: Proceedings of the National Conference* eds. J. F. Kavanagh and T. J. Truss. Parkton, MD: York Press.

Shaywitz, S. E., and Shaywitz, B. A. in press. Introduction to Symposium on Attention Deficit Disorder. *Journal of Learning Disabilities.*

Shaywitz, S. E., Schnell, C., Shaywitz, B. A., and Towle, V. R. 1986. Yale children's inventory (YCI): An instrument to assess children with attention deficits and learning disabilities I. Scale development and psychometric properties. *Journal of Abnormal Child Psychology* 14:347–64.

Shaywitz, S. E., Shaywitz, B. A., McGraw, K., and Groll, S. 1984. Current status of the neuromaturational examination as an index of learning disability. *Journal of Pediatrics* 104:819–25.

Shaywitz, S. E., Shaywitz, B. A., Schnell, C., and Towle, V. R. 1988. Concurrent and predictive validity of the Yale Children's Inventory: An instrument to assess children with attentional deficits and learning disabilities. *Pediatrics* 81:562–71.

Skinner, H. A. 1981. Toward the integration of classification theory and methods. *Journal of Abnormal Psychology* 90:68–87.

Studdert-Kennedy, M., and Shankweiler, D. 1970. Hemispheric specialization for speech perception. *Journal of the Acoustical Society of America* 48:579–94.

Taylor, H. G., Satz, P., and Friel, J. 1979. Developmental dyslexia in relation to other childhood reading disorders: Significance and clinical utility. *Reading Research Quarterly* 15:84–101.

Valencia, R. R., Henderson, R. W., and Rankin, R. J. 1985. Family status, family constellation, and home environmental variables as predictors of cognitive performance of Mexican-American children. *Journal of Educational Psychology* 77:323–31.

Vellutino, F. R. 1979. *Dyslexia: Theory and Research.* Cambridge, MA: MIT Press.

Wechsler, D. 1974. *Wechsler Intelligence Scale for Children–Revised.* New York: The Psychological Corporation.

Wiederholt, J. L. 1986. *Formal Reading Inventory: A Method of Assessing Silent Reading Comprehension and Oral Reading Miscues.* Austin, TX: Pro-Ed.

Wiederholt, J. L., and Bryant, B. R. 1986. *Gray Oral Reading Test—Revised.* Austin, TX: Pro-Ed.

Wolf, M. 1981. The word-retrieval process and reading in children and aphasics. In *Children's Language* (Vol. 3), ed. K. Nelson. New York: Gardner Press.

Woodcock, R. W., and Johnson, M. B. 1977. *Woodcock–Johnson Psychoeducational Battery.* Hingham, MA: Teaching Resources Corporation.

Chapter • 3

Colorado Reading Project
An Update

J. C. DeFries, R. K. Olson, B. F. Pennington, and S. D. Smith

In 1984 the National Institute of Child Health and Human Development (NICHD) sponsored a conference entitled "Biobehavioral Measures of Dyslexia." In a preface to the published proceedings of this conference, Gray and Kavanagh (1985) noted that: "Because the NICHD is currently supporting one collaborative interdisciplinary research project with a focus on reading, the Colorado Reading Project, this project served as one of the cornerstones for the development of the conference (p. x)." Since 1979, research at the University of Colorado concerning the etiology of reading disability had been supported in part by a program project grant from the NICHD. During the NICHD conference, co-investigators associated with the Colorado Reading Project summarized results obtained during its first five years. DeFries (1985) reviewed the background of the Colorado Reading Project and presented results of family, longitudinal, and risk analyses. Olson (1985) evaluated the component processes in reading and spelling, especially with regard to phonological and orthographic coding deficits in reading-disabled children. Decker and Vandenberg (1985) reviewed preliminary data obtained from a twin study of reading disability, and Shucard et al. (1985) described findings obtained from electrophysiological studies of cerebral functional specialization in disabled and normal readers.

This work was supported in part by a program project grant from the NICHD (HD-11681). We wish to acknowledge the invaluable contributions of staff members of the many Colorado school districts and of the families who participated in the study.

To date, the Colorado Reading Project has received continuous NICHD support for over ten years. The long-range objectives of this program project remain the identification, characterization, and validation of distinct subtypes or dimensions of reading disability. To accomplish these objectives, a test battery that includes measures of cognitive abilities and of reading and language processes is being administered to a sample of identical and fraternal twin pairs in which at least one member of each pair is reading disabled, to parents of these twins, to members of identical and fraternal twin families in which the children are normal readers, and to a longitudinal sample of nontwin reading-disabled and control children. Resulting twin and family data are being used to validate alternative typologies or dimensions of reading disability and to conduct genetic, longitudinal, and risk analyses. In addition, a survey of immune disorders and laterality is being administered to the twin sample, and data from program project families who manifest apparent autosomal dominance for reading disability are being subjected to linkage analysis using state-of-the-art genetic markers, including DNA restriction fragment length polymorphisms.

For administrative and logistical convenience, the Colorado Reading Project currently includes four substantive components: Twin/Family Study; Reading and Language Processes; Epidemiology of Immunological Differences; and Linkage Analysis. The primary objective of the present report is to summarize the results of recent research conducted within each of these components.

TWIN/FAMILY STUDY

In order to assess the genetic etiology of reading disability, a twin study was initiated in 1982 as part of the Colorado Reading Project. Administrators and school personnel in a total of 27 different school districts within the State of Colorado currently participate in this study. Without regard to reading status, all twin pairs within each district are identified and permission is then sought from parents to review the school records of both members of each pair for evidence of reading problems. If either member of a twin pair manifests a positive history of reading problems (e.g., low reading achievement test scores, referral to a reading therapist because of poor reading performance, reports by classroom teachers or school psychologists, etc.), both members of the pair are invited to complete an extensive battery of tests in our laboratories at the Institute for Behavioral Genetics and Department of Psychology, University of Colorado, Boulder.

In the laboratory of J. C. DeFries, an extensive psychometric test battery that includes the Wechsler Intelligence Scale for Children–

Revised (WISC–R; Wechsler 1974) or the Wechsler Adult Intelligence Scale–Revised (WAIS–R; Wechsler 1981) and the Peabody Individual Achievement Test (PIAT; Dunn and Markwardt 1970) is administered to the twins. In the laboratory of R. K. Olson, a battery of tests, including measures of phonological and orthographic coding, experimental measures of word recognition and reading comprehension, and measures of eye movements, is also administered to both members of each twin pair. Employing discriminant weights estimated from an analysis of PIAT Reading Recognition, Reading Comprehension, and Spelling data obtained from an independent sample of 140 reading-disabled and 140 control nontwin children (DeFries 1985), a discriminant function score is then computed for each subject. In order for an individual to be diagnosed as reading disabled in this component of the program project, the person must have a positive school history for reading problems and also be classified as affected by the discriminant score. Additional diagnostic criteria include an IQ score of at least 90 on either the Verbal or Performance Scale of the WISC or WAIS; no evidence of neurological, emotional, or behavioral problems; and no uncorrected visual or auditory acuity deficits.

A comparison group of control twins is also tested. Control twin pairs are matched to probands on the basis of age, gender, and school district. In order for a twin pair to be included in the control sample, both members of the pair must have a negative school history for reading problems and at least one member must be classified as unaffected by the discriminant analysis.

Selected items from the Nichols and Bilbro (1966) questionnaire are used to determine zygosity of same-sex twin pairs. In ambiguous cases, zygosity of the pair is confirmed by analysis of blood samples. As of December 31, 1989, a total of 99 pairs of identical (monozygotic, or MZ) twins, 73 pairs of same-sex fraternal (dizygotic, or DZ) twins, and 39 pairs of opposite-sex DZ twins meet our criteria for inclusion in the proband sample (i.e., at least one member of the pair of twins is reading disabled). In addition, a total of 99 pairs of MZ twins, 68 pairs of same-sex DZ twins, and 16 pairs of opposite-sex DZ twins compose the current control sample. These twins ranged in age from 8 to 20 years at the time of testing and all were reared in English-speaking, middle-class homes.

In contrast to the referred sample of nontwin reading-disabled children in which the gender ratio was 3.8 males to each female (DeFries 1985), the numbers of reading-disabled males and females in the current twin sample are 147 and 153, respectively. Because female MZ pairs tend to be overrepresented in twin studies (Lykken, Tellegen, and DeRubeis 1978), this lower gender ratio for reading-disabled members of twin pairs included in the Colorado Reading Project may be due in part to a differential volunteer rate of male and female twin pairs. In accordance with this expectation, the gender ratio in the sample of MZ probands is somewhat lower than that for DZ probands: 68 MZ males, 84 MZ females, 79 DZ males, and 69 DZ females. However, neither gender ratio deviates substantially from equality (viz., 0.81 versus 1.15, respectively). In addition, Vogel (1990) notes that referred samples of learning-disabled children may not be representative of learning-disabled children in the general population. Thus, the excess of male subjects invariably found in system-identified populations of reading-disabled children may be due at least in part to a referral bias.

Twin Concordance Rates

Previous twin studies of reading disability (Zerbin-Rüdin 1967; Bakwin 1973; Stevenson et al. 1987) employed a comparison of concordance rates as a test for genetic etiology. Although the concordance rate for MZ twin pairs exceeded that for DZ pairs in each of these three relatively small studies (14–31 pairs of MZ twins and 27–42 pairs of DZ twins), substantial variation in concordance rates occurred among the studies. Results obtained by Zerbin-Rüdin (1967) and Bakwin (1973) suggest that reading deficits may be highly heritable, whereas those of Stevenson et al. (1987) indicate substantially less genetic influence. (For a more detailed review of previous twin studies of reading disability and the estimation of concordance rates, see DeFries and Gillis in press.)

The number of reading-disabled twin pairs tested to date in the Colorado Reading Project exceeds the total number of affected pairs in all previous studies. Therefore, the results of this single study warrant considerable confidence. The probandwise concordance rate for 99 MZ twin pairs tested in the Colorado Reading Project is 70%, whereas that for 112 DZ twin pairs is 48%. These results confirm the evidence for at least some genetic etiology of reading disability obtained in previous twin studies.

Multiple Regression Analysis of Twin Data

Although a comparison of concordance rates as a test for genetic etiology is appropriate for categorical variables such as presence or absence of an illness, reading disability is operationally defined (Wong 1986; Stevenson et al. 1987) and its diagnosis is made on the basis of arbitrary cut-off points along a continuous dimension (e.g., reading performance). Transformation of a continuous measure into a categorical variable (e.g., reading disabled versus normal) obviously results in a loss of information pertaining to the continuum of variation in reading performance.

DeFries and Fulker (1985) recently proposed a methodology that facilitates an analysis of the etiology of deviant scores as well as individual differences within the proband group. In contrast to a comparison of concordance rates in MZ and DZ twin pairs, a comparison of MZ and DZ cotwin means was advocated as a test for genetic etiology. As illustrated in figure 1, when probands have been ascertained because of deviant scores on a continuous measure such as reading perfor-

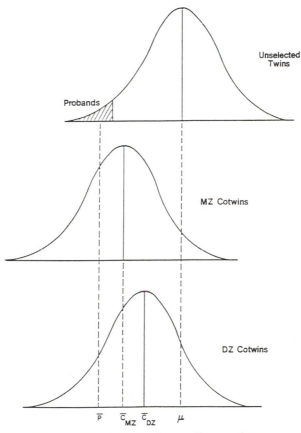

Figure 1. Hypothetical distributions for reading performance of an unselected sample of twins, and of the identical (MZ) and fraternal (DZ) cotwins of probands with a reading disability. The differential regression of the MZ and DZ cotwin means toward the mean of the unselected population (μ) provides a test of genetic etiology. From Evidence for a Genetic Aetiology in Reading Disability of Twins by J. C. DeFries, D. W. Fulker, and M. C. LaBuda, 1987, *Nature* 329:537. Copyright 1987 by Macmillan Journals Ltd. Reprinted by permission.

mance, the scores of both the MZ and DZ cotwins are expected to regress toward the mean of the unselected population. To the extent that
the condition has a genetic etiology, however, this regression toward
the mean should differ for MZ and DZ cotwins. Because members of
MZ twin pairs are genetically identical, whereas members of DZ pairs
share only about one-half of their segregating genes on average, scores
of DZ cotwins should regress more toward the mean of the unselected
population. Thus, if the MZ and DZ proband means are equal, a t-test
of the difference between the means of the MZ and DZ cotwins would
provide a test for genetic etiology. However, the partial regression of
cotwin's score on the coefficient of relationship ($R = 1.0$ for MZ twin
pairs and 0.5 for DZ twin pairs), independent of proband's score, provides a more general, statistically powerful, and flexible test (DeFries
and Fulker 1985, 1988).

Two regression models were formulated: (1) a basic model in which
the partial regression of cotwin's score on the coefficient of relationship
provides a test for genetic etiology; and (2) an augmented model that
also contains an interaction term between proband's score and relationships. These two models are as follows:

$$C = B_1P + B_2R + A \qquad (1)$$

and

$$C = B_3P + B_4R + B_5PR + A, \qquad (2)$$

where C is the cotwin's score, P is the proband's score, R is the coefficient of relationship, and PR is the product of proband's score and relationship. Because inclusion of the interaction term in the augmented
model changes the expectations for the partial regression coefficients
estimated from the basic model, the coefficients of P and R have different subscripts in equations 1 and 2.

DeFries and Fulker (1985) showed that B_1, the partial regression of
cotwin's score on proband's score, is a measure of average MZ and DZ
twin resemblance, whereas B_2 equals twice the difference between the
means for MZ and DZ cotwins after covariance adjustment for any difference between scores of MZ and DZ probands. Thus, B_2 was advocated as a test of significance for genetic etiology. In addition, they
demonstrated that B_3 and B_5 yield direct estimates of the proportion of
variance due to environmental influences shared by members of twin
pairs (c^2) and heritability (h^2), respectively.

DeFries and Fulker (1985) also noted that the results of fitting the
basic model to selected twin data could be used to obtain an estimate of
h^2_g, a measure of the extent to which the deficit of probands is due to
heritable influences. In addition, it was suggested that a comparison of
h^2_g and h^2 could be employed to test the hypothesis that the etiology of

extreme scores differs from that of variation within the normal range. Whereas the deficit of probands could be due to a major gene effect or to some gross environmental insult, for example, individual differences within the selected group might be due to multifactorial influences. If the etiology of deviant scores differs from that of variation within the normal range, h^2_g and h^2 would be expected to differ in magnitude. However, if probands merely represent the lower tail of a normal distribution of individual differences, h^2_g and h^2 should be of similar magnitude. More recently, DeFries and Fulker (1988) showed that a simple transformation of twin data (each score is expressed as a deviation from the mean of the unselected population and then divided by the difference between the proband and control means) prior to regression analysis facilitates a direct test of the hypothesis that the etiology of extreme scores differs from that of individual differences within the normal range. When MZ and DZ twin data are transformed in this simple manner, $B_2 = h^2_g$ and B_4 provides a significance test for $h^2_g - h^2$.

Because the probands in the Colorado Reading Project were selected on the basis of their discriminant scores (a composite measure of reading performance), the basic and augmented models were fitted to data for that measure. The average discriminant scores of the MZ and DZ probands and cotwins, expressed as standardized deviations from the control mean, are presented in table I. (Data from concordant twin pairs have been double entered for all analyses in a manner analogous to that used for computation of probandwise concordance rates.) From this table it may be seen that the average discriminant scores of the MZ and DZ probands are highly similar and over three standard deviations below the mean of the comparison sample of unaffected twins. In addition, it may be seen that the scores of the MZ cotwins have regressed only 0.25 standard deviation units on the average toward the control mean, whereas those of the DZ cotwins have regressed 0.95 standard deviation units. When the basic model was fitted to these data, $B_2 = -1.47 \pm 0.33$ ($p < .001$, one tailed). This highly significant coefficient is a function of the differential regression of the MZ and DZ cotwin scores and provides the best evidence to date for the heritable nature of reading disability.

Table I. Mean Discriminant Score of 99 Pairs of Identical Twins and 112 Pairs of Fraternal Twins in Which at Least One Member of Each Pair is Reading Disabled

	Probands	Cotwins
Identical	− 3.13	− 2.88
Fraternal	− 3.05	− 2.10

Note: Scores are expressed as standardized deviations from the mean score of 366 control twins.

In order to estimate h^2_g, the basic model was fitted to transformed discriminant function data. Because the means of identical and fraternal probands differ slightly, different transformations were employed for these two groups. When the basic model was fitted to these transformed data, $h^2_g = 0.47 \pm 0.11$ ($p < .001$). This highly significant parameter estimate suggests that about one-half of the reading performance deficit of probands, on average, is due to heritable influences.

When the augmented model was fitted to these transformed discriminant function data, $B_5 = h^2 = 0.73 \pm 0.36$ ($p < .01$, one tailed) and $B_3 = c^2 = 0.11 \pm 0.27$ ($p > .25$). These results suggest that individual differences within the selected group are highly heritable, whereas environmental influences that are shared by members of twin pairs are not an important source of variation. Moreover, although the estimates of h^2 and h^2_g are rather discrepant (0.73 and 0.47, respectively), suggesting that probands may not merely represent the lower tail of a normal distribution of individual differences, the difference between these two parameter estimates is not significant ($B_4 = -0.26 \pm 0.38$, $p > .25$).

Statistical Power

The multiple regression analysis of selected twin data provides a statistically powerful test of genetic etiology (DeFries and Fulker 1988). For example, when the basic model was fitted to transformed discriminant function data from the present sample of reading-disabled probands and cotwins, the estimate for $B_2 = h^2_g = 0.47$. The corresponding squared multiple correlation is 0.26, and the correlation between proband and cotwin scores is 0.43. Thus, the power (Cohen 1977) to detect a significant B_2 at the 0.05 level (one-tailed test) in a sample of 100 pairs of MZ and 100 pairs of DZ twins is 0.99.

Although the multiple regression test for genetic etiology is statistically powerful, the probability of rejecting the null hypothesis that $B_5 = h^2 = 0.0$ is no greater than that for estimates obtained from alternative twin analyses. For example, given the present data set in which $h^2 = 0.73$ and the corresponding squared multiple correlation (0.27), the power to detect a significant h^2 at the 0.05 level (one-tailed test) in a sample of 100 pairs of MZ and 100 pairs of DZ twins is 0.49. In a sample of 200 pairs of MZ and 200 pairs of DZ twins, the power increases to a more respectable 0.73.

Because the power to detect a significant h^2 is relatively low, the power to detect a significant difference between h^2_g and h^2 will be even lower. Given the data in the present sample in which $h^2_g = 0.47$ and $h^2 = 0.73$ and the associated squared multiple correlations, the power to detect a significant $B_4 = h^2_g - h^2$ at the 0.05 level (two-tailed test because there is no a priori expectation regarding the direction of the difference) in a sample of 200 pairs of MZ and 200 pairs of DZ twins is less than 0.20. Thus, a larger sample of twins will be required to test more rigorously the hypothesis that the etiology of extreme scores differs from that of individual differences within the normal range. However, because such a test is of considerable interest, especially with regard to the issue of the specificity of the deficit in reading disability (Foorman 1989), additional testing of twins in the Colorado Reading Project is clearly warranted.

Differential Etiology

The multiple regression analysis of selected twin data is also a highly flexible methodology. The basic and augmented models can be easily extended to include other main effects and interactions (Cohen and Cohen 1975) to test for differential genetic and environmental influences (DeFries and Gillis in press; Olson et al. in press-a). Because the multiple regression test for genetic etiology is statistically powerful, the test for differential genetic etiology is also relatively powerful. For example, if h^2_g in two subtypes differed by 0.5, the power to detect a significant interaction between R and subtype at the 0.05 level (two-tailed test) in a sample of 100 pairs of MZ and 100 pairs of DZ twins would be about 0.75 (DeFries and Fulker 1988). If the difference in h^2_g between subtypes were only 0.3, the power would be only about 0.3. However, by increasing the sample size to 150 pairs of MZ twins and 150 pairs of DZ twins, the power would be increased to about 0.90 and 0.50 in these two cases.

Wadsworth, Gillis, and DeFries (1990) recently employed this methodology to test a hypothesis that the genetic etiology of reading disability may differ as a function of age (Stevenson et al. 1987). When the basic model was fitted separately to data from younger (8.3–14.0 years) and older (14.1–20.2) twin pairs, estimates of h^2_g were 0.49 ± 0.12 and 0.39 ± 0.24, respectively. Thus, these results are consistent with the hypothesis of Stevenson et al. (1987) that genetic factors may be less important as a cause of reading disability in older children. However, the difference between these two estimates was found to be nonsignificant ($p > .50$) when an extension of the basic model that included an interaction between group membership and relationship was fitted simultaneously to data from both the younger and older twin pairs. Application of a more powerful test of differential genetic etiology that included age and its interactions as continuous measures in a regression model also yielded a nonsignificant ($p > .50$) result. When the basic model was fitted to data from twin pairs divided into three age groups (8.3–12.5, 12.6–15.5, and 15.6–20.2 years), resulting estimates of h^2_g were 0.48 ± 0.13, 0.26 ± 0.20, and 0.76 ± 0.40. Although this result suggests that genetic factors may be less important as a cause of reading problems during adolescence, a test for differential genetic etiology as a quadratic function of age was also nonsignificant. Thus, a more rigorous test of the hypothesis that the genetic etiology of reading disability differs as a function of age must also await the testing of additional twins in the Colorado Reading Project.

READING AND LANGUAGE PROCESSES

The focus of this component of the Colorado Reading Project is specific reading processes and related perceptual and language skills. The major goals are to evaluate profiles of component reading and language skills in reading-disabled and normal groups, to describe the range of individual differences within the reading-disabled population, and to assess the relative influence of genetic and environmental influences on deficits in specific reading processes and related cognitive skills. Progress in achieving these goals will be reviewed in three sub-sections. First, performance profiles will be compared for groups of younger normal readers and older disabled readers matched on level of word recognition. Second, the genetic etiologies of deficits in two specific components of word recognition will be compared. Third, differential genetic etiology of word-recognition deficits will be evaluated in relation to several subtype variables.

Disabled and Normal Profiles

Are there significant differences between disabled and normal readers' profiles of component reading and language skills, or are disabled readers equally depressed on all component reading and language skills? When disabled readers are compared with same-age normal readers, it is not surprising to find that the disabled readers are significantly lower on all reading and related skills. A number of researchers have argued that a more appropriate comparison of profile differences between disabled and normal readers can be obtained by matching older disabled and younger normal groups on a measure of reading (cf. Bryant and Goswami 1986).

Our reading-level-match comparisons of disabled and normal groups have used the PIAT word recognition test as the matching variable. From this reference point, it was found that the older disabled group ($M = 15.6$ years) was significantly better than the younger normal group (M = 10.4 years) on measures of reading comprehension (Conners and Olson in press). Results obtained from path analyses indicated that the disabled readers' superior performance on reading comprehension was related to their superior performance (in raw scores) on the Wechsler (1974, 1981) verbal subtests. Thus, by relying on their greater absolute level of verbal intelligence, the older disabled readers' comprehension of written text was better than would be expected from their very low ability in isolated word recognition. However, the disabled subjects' uniquely poor word recognition skills constrained their reading comprehension to levels substantially below that of normal readers at the same age and IQ.

The basis for disabled readers' poor word recognition has been a central focus of our research. Tasks were designed to measure subjects' skills in two component processes of word recognition, phonological coding, and orthographic coding (Olson et al. 1989). The phonological coding task required subjects to read aloud 85 nonwords of varying difficulty (e.g., int, tegwop, calch) as quickly and accurately as possible. The subject's score in this task was a composite of z scores for accuracy and speed on correct responses. Phonological coding is particularly important when readers encounter unfamiliar printed words. Recent evidence has indicated that phonological coding processes are also involved in the skilled reading of familiar words (Van Orden 1987).

The second component process in word recognition, orthographic coding, was measured by having subjects designate the word in 80 word-pseudohomophone pairs (e.g., rain, rane; salmon, sammon) as quickly as possible. The two letter strings in each pair were phonologically identical (i.e., they would sound the same if pronounced according to common phonological rules). Therefore, subjects had to recognize the specific orthographic pattern for the target word to make a correct choice. Scores on this task were based on the subject's combined z scores for accuracy and speed on correct responses. Orthographic coding is a particularly important process in reading English, which contains many homophones that must be discriminated (e.g., their, there), and many "exception" words that do not conform to common phonological rules (e.g., yacht, said). The theoretical background for the orthographic and phonological tasks is discussed in Olson et al. (in press-b).

When the older reading-disabled and younger normal groups matched on PIAT word recognition were compared on the phonological and orthographic tasks, a striking difference in profiles was observed (Olson et al. 1989). The disabled readers' performance on the orthographic task was slightly, but significantly, better than that of the younger normal group. In contrast, the disabled readers' performance on the phonological coding task was 0.78 of a standard deviation below the mean for the younger normal group ($p < .01$). Thus, on average, disabled readers had phonological coding skills that were well below the levels expected from their word recognition.

These results replicated findings from an earlier study in the Colorado Reading Project that used different samples and measures of phonological and orthographic coding (Olson et al. 1985). However, the results of reading-level-match studies from other laboratories have been less consistent. Some have found a phonological deficit in disabled readers (cf. Snowling 1980), whereas others have reported that disabled readers' phonological coding was not significantly different from that of younger normal readers at the same level of word recognition (cf. Treiman and Hirsh-Pasek 1985). A recent meta analysis of reading-level-match studies on phonological coding concluded that most of the null results could be accounted for by factors such as ceiling effects, regression artifacts in sample selection, and inadequate assessment and control of IQ differences between the groups (Olson et al. in press-b; Rack, Snowling, and Olson submitted).

The best evidence indicates that most children who meet the usual selection criteria for specific reading disability have a unique problem in phonological coding. However, our disabled readers showed substantial within-group variance in phonological coding after adjustment for their level of word recognition. Much of this variance was related to the disabled readers' performance on a "pig latin" task that required segmental language skills. Disabled readers who were relatively good at this segmental language task were also relatively good in phonological coding (Conners and Olson in press).

The disabled readers' phonological coding was also related to within-group variance in verbal IQ. Earlier results from the Colorado Reading Project revealed a small, but significant, *negative* partial correlation ($r = -.28$, $N = 59$) between disabled readers' accuracy in oral nonword reading and their combined scores on four Wechsler subtests (Information, Vocabulary, Similarities, and Comprehension) that were included in Kaufman's (1975) verbal factor (Olson et al. 1985). (The partialed variable was PIAT word recognition.) Rack and Olson (1989) found a similar negative partial correlation ($r = -.29$, $N = 218$) between our current phonological coding measure and Kaufman's verbal factor in a much larger sample. These small negative correlations suggest that factors associated with low verbal intelligence may be contributing to low word recognition for some disabled readers in our sample. But for most disabled readers, poor phonological coding and related segmental language skills seem to be the major constraints on their development of word recognition. Behavioral genetic analyses reviewed in the following section indicate that disabled readers' heritable deficits in word recognition are strongly related to their heritable deficits in phonological coding.

Behavioral Genetic Analyses

The genetic etiology of disabled readers' deficits in word recognition, phonological coding, and orthographic coding was examined by Olson et al. (1989) using the regression model developed by DeFries and Fulker (1985). The difference between MZ and DZ cotwins' regression toward the normal mean yielded an estimate of the degree to which the probands' group deficit was heritable (h^2_g). When the basic model (equation 1) was fitted to word recognition data from 117 twin pairs, h^2_g = 0.40 ± 0.12, ($p < .01$), indicating that about 40% of the probands' deficit was due to heritable influences. Corresponding estimates of h^2_g for phonological and orthographic coding deficits were 0.47 ± 0.14 and 0.28 ± 0.16, respectively. Thus, the phonological coding deficits of reading-disabled children are significantly heritable, whereas their orthographic coding deficits are not.

Additional analyses assessed the genetic covariance between subjects' deficits in word recognition and their deficits in phonological and orthographic coding (Olson et al. 1989). Genetic covariance is an index of the degree to which genetic variance in one variable is shared with that in another variable (Plomin, DeFries, and McClearn 1990). Because subjects were selected for word-recognition deficits in this analysis, the h^2_g of correlated variables estimates the genetic covariance between word recognition and the correlated variable divided by their phenotypic covariance, i.e., a measure of the extent to which the observed association is due to genetic influence. Resulting estimates of h^2_g for phonological and orthographic coding were 0.93 ± 0.16, and −0.16 ± 0.27, respectively, suggesting a substantial genetic covariance between word recognition and phonological coding.

Our most recent unpublished analyses with a much larger sample (284 pairs of twins) confirm the above pattern of differential heritabilities and genetic covariance for word recognition, phonological coding, and orthographic coding. Estimates of h^2_g for word-recognition deficits (0.54 ± 0.08), phonological coding (0.54 ± 0.10), and orthographic coding (0.28 ± 0.11) are slightly higher than the previously reported estimates (Olson et al. 1989). For the genetic covariance analysis, a bivariate form of the basic model was employed in which the cotwins' scores for either phonological or orthographic coding were predicted from the word recognition scores of probands. The resulting "bivariate h^2_g" estimates the genetic covariance between word recognition and the correlated variable, divided by the phenotypic variance of word recognition. Thus, a comparison of the two bivariate h^2_g estimates involving phonological and orthographic coding provides a direct test of their differential genetic covariance with word recognition. As in our previous analyses, the bivariate h^2_g estimate between word recognition and phonological coding (0.81 ± 0.14) is substantially higher than between word recognition and orthographic coding (0.27 ± 0.18). The difference between these two estimates is statistically significant ($p < .05$) when tested in a LISREL model.

The above results clearly indicate a strong genetic influence on deficits in word recognition, primarily through heritable deficits in phonological coding. However, the path of genetic influence on phonological coding may ultimately be through heritable differences in segmental language skills. Olson et al. (1989) reported significant genetic covariance between deficits in phonological coding and the "pig-latin" task discussed earlier ($h^2_g = 0.81 \pm 0.38$), and between phonological coding and a rhyme-generation task ($h^2_g = 0.99 \pm 0.43$). Further research is underway to confirm this relation with additional measures of segmental language skills.

The low heritability and genetic covariance estimates for orthographic coding indicate that this skill is predominantly influenced by environmental factors. Stanovich and West (1989) found that indirect measures of reading experience accounted for significant variance in measures similar to our orthographic coding task, after partialing variance in phonological coding. Shared home and school environments for print exposure in our MZ and DZ twin pairs may thus be responsible for the significant c^2 (shared environment) estimates that we are finding for individual differences in orthographic coding (but not phonological coding) within the disabled and normal groups.

Differential Heritability of Word-Recognition Deficits

Our estimates of h^2_g for word recognition are estimates of the heritability for the *group* deficit. It is possible that there are systematic differences in h^2_g within the disabled group that are related to subtype variables. In the first section of this chapter there was a discussion of the differential heritability of disabled subjects' discriminant scores depending on age (Wadsworth, Gillis, and DeFries 1990). The same model used in that analysis has been applied to evaluate differences in h^2_g for word recognition as a function of deficit severity, phonological coding, orthographic coding, IQ, gender, and age (Olson et al. in press-a).

Severity of word-recognition deficits was the subject of our initial subtype analysis. There was a continuous distribution of word-recognition deficits below the cutoff score of one standard deviation

(*SD*) below the mean of the normal control group. Therefore, the significance test for differential h^2_g was based on its linear relation to the severity of word-recognition deficits. The test was statistically significant ($p = .045$). The magnitude and direction of this differential heritability was indicated by a separate assessment of h^2_g for groups divided at the mean word-recognition deficit of -2.4 *SD*. For 85 twin pairs whose proband was below the group mean deficit of -2.4 *SD* (subgroup mean $= -3.31$ *SD*), $h^2_g = 0.51 \pm 0.11$. For 105 pairs above the group mean deficit (subgroup mean $= -1.68$ *SD*), $h^2_g = 0.80 \pm 0.17$. These results thus indicate significantly higher heritability for *less* severe deficits in word recognition. We have examined the twins' birth and medical information provided by the parents to determine if environmental insults might have lead to the more severe deficits in word recognition. Birth and medical problems were rare and their prevalence was not significantly different between the more and less severe subgroups (Olson et al. in press-a). We are now exploring other possible explanations for the differential etiology of more and less severe reading deficits.

The above differences in h^2_g as a function of deficit severity in word recognition complicate the analysis of other subtype variables that are correlated with word recognition. Therefore, we adjusted the orthographic coding, phonological coding, and IQ variables for their relation to word recognition before using those variables as subtype dimensions. Differential h^2_g of word recognition as a function of differences in phonological coding (adjusted for word recognition) approached statistical significance ($p = .057$). For 86 pairs who were lower than the mean adjusted phonological coding score, $h^2_g = 0.74 \pm 0.15$. For 104 pairs above the mean, $h^2_g = 0.54 \pm 0.11$. Thus, subjects who were relatively poor phonological coders, compared to their word recognition, tended to have higher heritabilities for their deficits in word recognition. This result is consistent with the high genetic covariance between word recognition and phonological coding that was discussed earlier. Environmental factors such as reading experience may play a greater role in the word-recognition deficits of the better phonological coders.

None of the other subtype variables approached statistical significance for predicting differential h^2_g of disabled readers' word recognition. However, there was an interesting trend in relation to IQ. After phonological coding, the next highest level of statistical significance for differential h^2_g involved full-scale IQ ($p = .17$). For this analysis, 30 twin pairs who did not meet the minimum verbal or performance IQ criterion of 90 were added to the sample to increase the IQ range. For 123 pairs whose mean IQ was 91, $h^2_g = 0.40 \pm 0.10$. For 124 pairs whose mean IQ was 107, $h^2_g = 0.67 \pm 0.11$. This trend suggests that the heritability for word-recognition deficits is higher for subjects whose IQ is high relative to their word recognition ability. Although the word-recognition deficits of subjects with lower IQ are significantly heritable, environmental influences may be relatively more important as a cause of reading disability in these subjects. Confirmation of these trends and marginally significant results for differential h^2_g will require a larger twin sample.

In summary, the behavioral genetic analyses in the Reading and Language Processes component of the Colorado Reading Project have yielded evidence for a significant genetic covariance between word-recognition deficits and phonological coding. In contrast, the relationship between word recognition and orthographic coding appears to be due largely to environmental influences. New measures of segmental language skills, visual processes, and reading experience have recently been added to the test battery to explore further the origins of genetic and environmental influences on word recognition and its component coding skills.

EPIDEMIOLOGY OF IMMUNOLOGICAL DIFFERENCES

The focus of this component of the Colorado Reading Project is on the clinical correlates of reading disability (dyslexia) and their relation to its etiology. Like other complex behavioral disorders, reading disability has a number of clinical correlates, some with a straightforward relation to its primary symptoms and others not so straightforward. One of the goals of research on subtypes of reading disability is to determine which putative clinical correlates are causally related either to reading disability in general or to one of its subtypes. The twin method employed in the Colorado Reading Project provides a powerful method of testing the validity of such subtypes defined in terms of clinical correlates. Specifically, the twin method permits several different validity tests, including tests of differential genetic etiology, genetic covariance, and cross-concordance.

For example, if subtypes are defined dichotomously (such as dyslexics with and without attention deficit hyperactivity disorder–ADHD), then the extended regression model described in the Twin/Family Study section of this chapter can provide a direct test for the differential genetic etiology of reading deficits in the two subtypes (see also LaBuda, DeFries, and Pennington 1990; Olson et al. in press-a). If differential heritability is found, that result validates the typology because it suggests differential genetic etiology for each subtype. Null results, as usual, are not conclusive because they may result from lack of power or from genetically distinct mechanisms (e.g., polygenic versus recessive) that are nonetheless essentially equal in their heritability.

If the subtype is defined using a continuous measure (such as ratings of ADHD), then the genetic covariance between reading measures and the continuous measure of the comorbid condition can be evaluated. This analysis provides an indirect estimate of whether there is a genetic correlation between the two dimensions. If the results are significant, then there is evidence that the same genetic factors influence both dimensions of performance. For instance, the results of Olson et al. (1989) indicate that there is a significant genetic covariance between word-recognition deficits and phonological coding, and that there is a common genetic etiology for reading disability and what many regard as its proximal cause, a deficit in phonological coding.

Cross-concordance analyses address the issue of genetic correlation using categorical measures, such as presence or absence of RD or ADHD, and can be applied either to the sample as a whole or to a subset of probands who have both disorders (e.g., RD + ADHD). When applied to the whole sample, a cross-concordance analysis examines whether the rates of the second disorder (e.g., ADHD) are significantly higher in the MZ versus DZ cotwins of probands who have the first disorder (e.g., RD). If so, there is evidence in the sample as a whole for a common etiology for the two disorders. The result of this analysis could conceivably differ from the result of the genetic covariance analysis discussed above, since the etiology of extreme scores on a dimension may vary from the etiology of variation on the whole dimension. Cross-concordance analysis of a subtype (e.g., RD + ADHD) examines the possibility that the disorders have a common etiology in a subtype, whether or not they do in the whole sample.

Clinical correlates of reading disability ostensibly include immune disorders (Geschwind and Behan 1982, 1984). We tested this apparent association in our extended family linkage sample and (to our surprise) replicated it (Pennington et al. 1987). Specifically, we found increased rates of both autoimmune and allergic disorders, but not comparison disorders (stuttering, migraines, or diagnosed ADHD), in familial dyslexics relative to the prevalence of these disorders in either non-dyslexic relatives or in the general population. However, we failed to find any association between dyslexia and non-right handedness, contrary to the neurobiological theory proposed by Geschwind and Galaburda (1985). Since the extended family linkage sample is a highly selected sample of dyslexic families (large, extended dyslexic families with a three-generation history of dyslexia—see Linkage Analysis section below), we felt it was important to assess the association between reading disability and immune disorders in a more representative population. Accordingly, we obtained data on the rates of immune and comparison disorders in the families of twins tested in the Colorado Reading Project. The use of twin samples also permitted a direct test of the cross-concordance of reading disability and immune disorders.

To examine the relation between reading disability and immune disorders in the twin samples, we obtained self-report data on immune and comparison disorders by mail questionnaires from 176 reading-disabled (RD) and 113 control twin families. These samples represent 83% and 66% of the program project samples, respectively. Rates for these disorders for individuals in RD versus control families and for RD versus non-RD individuals are given in table II. (These rates are adjusted for sex, since the sex ratios vary across groups; sex adjustment did not change the results.) As can be seen, these results appear to provide a clear non-replication of our earlier results. In fact, there were significantly higher rates of allergic disorders ($\chi^2 = 7.52$, $df = 1$, $p < .01$) and migraines ($\chi^2 = 5.46$, $df = 1$, $p < .05$) in the non-RD relatives of RD twins. These results suggest that an underlying factor could lead to reading disability in some relatives and to allergy or migraines in others, but it does not support the hypothesis that reading disability and immune disorders cosegregate in the same individuals. Either there is no cosegregation between reading disability and immune disorders or the cosegregation found earlier is true for only a small subtype of dyslexic families, which is not detectable in an analysis of the whole population. Another logical, but unlikely, possibility is that the association is present only in non-twin RD families.

To test the possibility of a subtype of dyslexia with immune disorders, we next examined the pairwise cross-concordance of reading dis-

Table II.   Immune Disorders and Reading Disability

	N	Immune Disorders			Comparison Disorders		
		Allergic	Asthma	Auto	Stutter	Hyper	Migraines
		Families					
RD Families (M/F = 1.05)	1044	20.1	9.2	5.3	2.5	2.0	9.2
Control Families (M/F = 0.90)	692	21.6	10.5	6.3	1.9	0.6	7.6
		Individuals					
RD (M/F = 1.05)	299	19.5	8.6	3.4	3.0	4.4	6.1
Non-RD Relatives (M/F = 0.95)	259	28.9**	10.3	3.6	2.4	1.3	11.2*
Non-RD Controls (M/F = 0.69)	325	23.8	10.7	4.6	1.5	0.8	8.1

* $p < .05$.
** $p < .01$.

ability and immune disorders in the twin samples. (Analyses employing probandwise concordance rates yielded similar results.) A genetic
etiology for reading disability already has been well established in this
sample (see Twin/Family Study section). Likewise, as shown in table
III, we found evidence for genetic etiology of atopic disorders (allergy
plus asthma), $\chi^2 = 28.19$ ($p < .001$). The critical question was whether
reading disability and atopic disorders were genetically correlated in all
or some of this sample. This issue was examined by computing the
cross-concordance in MZ versus DZ pairs, beginning with a proband
affected by reading disability and examining the rates of allergy/
asthma in the cotwins. Null results were obtained (table III), parallel-
ing the null results for the association of dyslexia and immune disorders in the entire twin sample. Likewise, null results were obtained
when we began with a proband with allergy/asthma and examined the
rates of dyslexia in the cotwin. We clearly rejected the hypothesis of
genetic correlation in the entire sample, but the hypothesis of a genetic
subtype remained to be tested.

In this analysis we selected twin probands who were affected with
both dyslexia and allergy/asthma and examined the cotwins' status for
both diagnoses (table IV). As can be seen, there is evidence for a genetic correlation in this subtype, because the MZ concordance rate for
this subtype is significantly higher than the DZ concordance rate.
However, since there are high rates of both dyslexia and self-reported
immune disorders in these samples, and since each of these disorders
is heritable, the significantly greater MZ concordance for the subtype
might be an artifact. We next performed a series of analyses to test this
possibility.

Several alternative methods may be employed to correct the twin
concordance rates for base rate. One method assumes population base
rates for dyslexia (e.g., 7.5%) and allergy/asthma (e.g., 13%), and uses
their cross-product to derive expectancies for having the two disorders

Table III. Concordance and Cross-Concordance of Allergy/Asthma in Total
Sample

	Number of Pairs	Concordant	Discordant
Pairwise Concordance of Allergy/Asthma in RD and Control Twins			
MZ	52	40 (0.77)	12 (0.33)
DZ	73	21 (0.29)	52 (0.71)
Pairwise Cross-Concordance of Reading Disability and Allergy			
MZ	59	20 (0.34)	39 (0.66)
DZ	41	16 (0.39)	25 (0.61)

Note: These are pairwise analyses. Similar results are obtained when probandwise analyses are performed.

Table IV.   Cross-Concordance of Reading Disability Plus Allergy/Asthma Subtype

	Pairs	Concordant	Discordant (1 + 2 + 3)
MZ	20	13 (0.65)	7 (0.35)
DZ	27	3 (0.11)	24 (0.89)
			$\chi^2 = 16.79, p < .001$

Note: Concordant = Both twins have RD and allergy/asthma; Discordant1 = one twin has both and the co-twin has RD but no allergy/asthma; Discordant2 = one twin has both and the co-twin has allergy/asthma but no RD; Discordant3 = one twin has both and the co-twin has neither allergy/asthma nor RD.

by chance alone. This gives a small expected frequency for RD with AD of roughly 1%, and, when applied to the data in table IV, results in a highly significant chi-square. If we use the higher base rates for the two conditions that we obtain from our control sample, the chi-square is still highly significant. The problem with these two types of correction is that they fail to account for the heritability of each condition, which leads to a higher expected percent of concordant MZs than concordant DZs.

The method that takes both population (for at least our sample) prevalence rates and heritabilities into consideration involves obtaining base rates for MZ and DZ concordances independently. Details of how to obtain these base rates are given in Gilger, Pennington, and DeFries (in review). These MZ and DZ concordance rates for reading disability were 60% and 46%, and for allergy/asthma they were 73% and 29%, respectively. Thus, if we assume that RD and AD are independently transmitted, then the expected MZ concordance for RD + AD equals 44% (60% × 73%). For DZs the expected concordance rate is 13%. Applying a chi-square goodness of fit analysis to the data in table IV reveals that the differences between observed and expected concordance rates are marginally significant ($\chi^2 = 3.66$, 1 df, $p < .07$). Further study of the observed frequencies in table IV shows that the significant chi-square is solely due to the fact that the MZ concordance rate is higher than expected if the two disorders are indeed independently heritable in the RD + AD proband twin pairs. The DZ rates are in fact identical to expectations. Given the manner by which expected values were calculated, we consider this test of differential concordances to be fairly conservative.

A remaining problem with our cross-concordance analysis is that currently it is based on a relatively small sample. Nevertheless, these preliminary results are convergent with preliminary results from the Linkage Analysis component indicating a subtype of familial dyslexia closely linked to the HLA region of chromosome 6, which contains many genes that affect the immune system. There may be a gene in this region that affects both reading and immune functions or, alternatively, there could be two closely linked genes that are independent in their pathophysiologies. Clearly more work is needed to validate the existence of a subtype of dyslexia associated with immune disorders and to understand the neurobiological mechanisms underlying this subtype.

LINKAGE ANALYSIS

Almost from the time reading disability first was described in the medical literature, early case reports and family studies led to the conclusion that it was inherited as an autosomal dominant condition (Hallgren 1950). More recent studies demonstrated that there probably is more than one mode of transmission (Finucci et al. 1976; Lewitter, DeFries, and Elston 1980), including autosomal dominant, autosomal recessive, and multifactorial inheritance. Localization and characterization of such genes would be of great value in understanding the mechanism of genetic influence on the reading process, which presumably could contribute to more effective therapy. Linkage analysis is a technique for localizing such genes along the chromosomes.

Linkage analysis has been used mainly to localize single major genes (often referred to as "Mendelian," in that the phenotypes are discrete and exhibit fairly clear recessive or dominant inheritance patterns), but the potential for localization of genes influencing quantitative traits has been recognized (Haseman and Elston 1972). With the advent of restriction fragment length polymorphisms (RFLPs) and the resulting explosion of markers all along the chromosomes, there has been increasing interest in using linkage analysis to examine conditions that may be due to more than one gene, either individually or in combination (Lander and Botstein 1986, 1989).

Linkage analysis is based on the fact that genes that are close together on the same chromosome tend to be inherited together as they are passed on from parent to child. Genes that are far apart on the same chromosome or on different chromosomes show random assortment as they are transmitted from generation to generation; that is, the probability that a child will inherit a specific allele is not influenced by the inheritance of the alleles at the other locus. If the inheritance pattern of the alleles from the two genes deviates significantly from random, this is taken as evidence that the genes are close together (linked). In practice, to localize a gene, its transmission is compared to the transmission of a battery of "marker" genes whose location is known; if linkage is found between the gene and one of the markers, the gene is localized to the chromosomal region of the marker. The distance between the gene and the marker can be estimated by the percentage of time the two alleles are not inherited together. This is termed recombination, and is due to crossing over between paired chromosomes in the region between the two loci. The frequency of recombination (expressed as θ) increases as the distance between genes increases. The probability that linkage exists, given a specific value of θ, can be expressed as a LOD score, the Log of the Odds of linkage. By convention, a LOD score greater than 3.0 is taken as evidence for linkage, and a LOD score less than -2.0 rejects linkage at that value of θ (Morton 1955). Evidence for genetic heterogeneity is obtained when linkage is demonstrated clearly in some families, but data from other families reject that linkage or support an alternate linkage (Morton 1956).

Previous linkage analysis with reading disability had suggested that it may be linked to the short arm/centromere heteromorphisms of chromosome 15 in some families (Smith et al. 1983). Subsequent studies have been designed to confirm that potential localization with DNA polymorphisms on chromosome 15, since these would provide additional and more easily replicated markers. Also, genetic heterogeneity was suspected, based on the wide range of the LOD scores from different families as well as theoretical expectations that a complex disability such as reading can be caused by more than one genetic factor. In addition to using statistical methods to test the LOD scores from chromosome 15 markers for homogeneity, markers from one other chromosome have been examined to see if there is suggestion of an alternate linkage, particularly in families clearly not showing linkage to chromosome 15. Based on pilot studies done using traditional genotyping markers, the Bf and GLO loci on chromosome 6 were chosen for further study. These loci are also intriguing since they are within the HLA region, which may have some bearing on the immunological variations suspected in disabled readers (Geschwind and Behan 1982; Pennington et al. 1986). A total of 22 families of children with reading disability has now been studied.

Present Sample

Families were selected from clinical populations in Denver and from the Colorado Reading Project. Initial selection criteria were an apparent extended family history of specific reading disability on one side of the family, following an apparent autosomal dominant pattern, and both biological parents and at least two children over 7 years of age available for study. All families were native English speaking and of middle-class background, and all family members in the study had a Verbal or Performance IQ of at least 90. A battery of tests was administered to each family member to confirm the history of the presence or absence of specific reading disability.

The definition of specific reading disability was the existence of significant difficulty in the tests measuring reading and spelling, with normal abilities in other academic areas. This diagnosis was made based on three factors: (1) Reading Quotient (RQ) (Finucci 1978); (2) the Specific Dyslexia Algorithm (SDA) as developed by Pennington, which specifies a pattern of high achievement in Mathematics and General Information, lower achievement in Reading Comprehension, and lowest in Reading Recognition and Spelling (Pennington et al. 1984); and (3) an early history of significant and persistent problems learning to read, without known etiology. From these criteria, five different categories were defined: affected (positive RQ or SDA and positive history); unaffected (negative RQ, SDA, and history); compensated (negative RQ and SDA, positive history); obligate carrier (negative RQ, SDA, and history, but with an affected child and affected sibling or parent); and questionable (anything other than the above; for example, positive RQ but negative history). For the linkage analysis, compensated individuals and obligate carriers were considered affected, and questionable individuals were omitted.

Blood samples were taken from all participating family members for typing of the traditional genotyping markers, chromosomal heteromorphisms, and DNA restriction fragment length polymorphisms. Informative family members have been typed for chromosomal variates and the DNA polymorphisms D15S1 (pDP151), D15S2 (pMS1-14), D15S3 (pJu201), D15S24 (CMW1), and TH114. Families were also typed and analyzed for three loci on chromosome 6: BF (properdin factor), GLO1 (glyoxylase I), and 2C5 (D6S8). Two forms of linkage analysis were performed: two-way, in which loci are examined two at a time; and multipoint, in which information from several markers is used simultaneously. The computer program LINKAGE (Lathrop et al. 1985) was used for these analyses, with reading disability represented as a fully penetrant, autosomal dominant, dichotomous trait. The resulting LOD scores were tested for homogeneity of the recombination fraction with HOMOG (Ott 1985).

Two-Way Analysis

The results of the two-way analysis with reading disability and chromosome 15 heteromorphisms are shown in table V. The maximum LOD score is 1.328 at a recombination level of 30%, which is inconclusive evidence for linkage. However, a wide range of LOD scores between families is observed, and, in particular, Family 6432 has a LOD score of 2.907 with no recombination. Since other families have clearly negative LOD scores, this suggests that heterogeneity may be present.

In testing for homogeneity of the LOD score data, the program

Table V. Linkage between SRD and Chromosome 15 Heteromorphisms

	Recombination Fraction				
	0.00	0.10	0.20	0.30	0.40
Family					
9007	$-\infty$	−0.389	−0.051	0.030	0.019
9008	$-\infty$	−0.267	−0.110	−0.049	−0.014
9102	$-\infty$	−0.957	−0.425	−0.168	−0.039
6372	$-\infty$	−0.350	0.164	0.276	0.201
6375	0.628	0.535	0.370	0.191	0.051
6432	**2.907**	**2.401**	**1.877**	**1.323**	**0.712**
6484	$-\infty$	−2.279	−0.750	−0.141	0.060
6491	$-\infty$	−1.331	−0.581	−0.227	−0.053
6576	0.514	0.328	0.175	0.070	0.015
8001	$-\infty$	−2.201	−1.114	−0.553	−0.215
8002	$-\infty$	−0.888	−0.297	−0.084	−0.014
8005	−1.703	−0.325	−0.119	−0.037	−0.006
8006	$-\infty$	−0.224	−0.057	−0.009	0.000
8007	0.301	0.255	0.204	0.146	0.079
8008	0.899	0.722	0.539	0.356	0.175
8010	$-\infty$	−0.253	−0.092	−0.036	−0.010
6371	0.602	0.465	0.318	0.170	0.049
1000	0.292	0.208	0.129	0.062	0.016
1001	$-\infty$	−0.229	−0.060	−0.011	−0.001
1002	0.292	0.208	0.129	0.062	0.016
442	$-\infty$	−0.425	−0.161	−0.043	0.003
Total	$-\infty$	−4.996	0.088	1.328	1.044

HOMOG utilizes two parameters, α and θ, to define three hypotheses: α is defined as the proportion of families showing linkage and θ is the recombination fraction. The null hypothesis, H_0, is that there is no linkage; α is set at 0 and θ at 0.5 (random assortment). The first alternate hypothesis (H_1) is that all of the families show linkage to the marker; α is set at 1.0 and θ is estimated from the data. The second alternate hypothesis is that heterogeneity exists; both α and θ are estimated from the data.

The results of this analysis are shown in table VI. For the hypothesis of heterogeneity, α was estimated to be 20%. The null hypothesis of no linkage can be rejected when compared to either of the alternate hypotheses. In addition, when the hypothesis of heterogeneity is compared to the hypothesis of homogeneous linkage, the hypothesis of homogeneity is just barely rejected ($P = 0.044$).

If there is heterogeneity, in that some families are linked and others are not, it is clear that summing LOD scores over all families is not valid. This means that the traditional criteria for acceptance of linkage, a total LOD score greater than 3, is not obtainable unless some external criteria can be found to subdivide families, or if analysis is restricted to

Table VI.   Test of Homogeneity (HOMOG; J. Ott): Reading Disability versus Chromosome 15 Heteromorphisms

H_0: No linkage ($\alpha = 0.00$, $\theta = 0.50$)
H_1: Linkage with homogeneity ($\alpha = 1.00$, $\theta = 0.30$)
H_2: Linkage with heterogeneity ($\alpha = 0.20$, $\theta = 0.00$)

	df	chi-square	p-value
H_2 vs. H_1	1	2.910	0.0440
H_1 vs. H_0	1	7.000	0.0041
H_2 vs. H_0	2	9.910	0.0035

very large families. Ott (1985) has suggested that, alternatively, the hypothesis of linkage may be accepted if the significance level for at least one of the three tests in HOMOG is significant at least at the 0.001 level. The results shown in table VI do not reach this criterion, since the *P* value for the most significant test (H_2 versus H_0) is 0.003.

Multipoint Analysis

The results of the multipoint analysis are shown in table VII. In addition to the chromosomal heteromorphisms, data from two DNA markers, TH114 and DP151, are included. These markers were the most informative and closest to the heteromorphisms of the DNA markers tested. The addition of DNA markers in a multipoint analysis of linkage supports, but does not add to, the overall LOD score or to the LOD score for Family 6432. When the test for homogeneity is performed with these data, the null hypothesis of no linkage cannot be rejected when compared to the hypothesis of linkage with homogeneity, but both the null hypothesis and the hypothesis of homogeneity are rejected when compared to the hypothesis of heterogeneity (table VIII). Again, however, the significance levels are not great enough to establish linkage without other confirming evidence. Thus, the results of both the two-way and multipoint linkage analyses do not confirm the existence of linkage, but do suggest that, if linkage exists, there is heterogeneity with only about 20% of the families showing linkage to chromosome 15.

Linkage results with markers from chromosome 6 were quite similar, but there were some interesting findings when these results were contrasted with the chromosome 15 data on a family-by-family basis. Again, the total LOD scores were not high (table IX); however, several families had LOD scores greater than 1.0, and Family 6432, which showed strong evidence for linkage to chromosome 15, shows negative linkage to chromosome 6 markers. In fact, families that tended to show stronger linkage to one chromosome tended to show less linkage to the

Table VII. Multipoint Linkage between SRD and Chromosome 15 Markers

Family		Markers and Map Position										
	0.4	0.3	0.2	0.1	15 centromere	0.075	0.15	0.225	TH114	0.03	0.07	DP151
9007	0.019	0.027	-0.056	-0.395	-17.917	-0.485	-0.081	0.054	-0.033	-0.127	-0.337	-∞
9008	-0.001	-0.027	-0.079	-0.224	-15.599	-0.296	-0.125	-0.095	-0.262	-0.370	-0.584	-1.511
9102	-0.040	-0.169	-0.429	-0.964	-32.035	-1.223	-0.693	-0.461	-0.517	-0.617	-0.840	-∞
6372	0.201	0.276	0.164	-0.350	-46.660	-0.614	0.030	0.295	0.410	0.423	0.434	0.444
6375	0.220	0.431	0.625	0.780	0.831	0.851	0.812	0.730	-∞	-0.290	-0.568	-∞
6432	**0.712**	**1.316**	**1.857**	**2.361**	**2.838**	**2.427**	**1.984**	**1.457**	**-0.233**	**0.821**	**0.826**	**-∞**
6484	0.058	-0.149	-0.769	-2.315	-∞	-3.084	-1.467	-0.853	-1.154	-1.488	-2.184	-∞
6491	-0.053	-0.227	-0.581	-1.331	-47.864	-1.727	-1.030	-0.813	-1.155	-1.403	-1.896	-∞
6576	0.015	0.070	0.175	0.328	0.514	0.372	0.247	0.144	0.070	0.060	0.051	0.042
8001	-0.214	-0.549	-1.107	-2.190	-49.853	-2.651	-1.519	-0.886	-0.450	-0.382	-0.316	-0.250
8002	-0.014	-0.084	-0.297	-0.888	-47.239	-1.155	-0.469	-0.183	-0.115	-0.130	-0.160	-0.211
8005	-0.006	-0.037	-0.119	-0.325	-1.703	-0.424	-0.197	-0.091	-0.037	-0.031	-0.025	-0.020
8006	0.000	-0.009	-0.057	-0.224	-15.647	-0.422	-0.256	-0.255	-0.480	-0.603	-0.834	-1.808
8007	0.059	0.098	0.120	0.127	0.118	0.028	-0.107	-0.347	-1.011	-1.312	-1.862	-∞
8008	0.175	0.356	0.539	0.722	0.899	0.747	0.576	0.361	-0.041	-0.198	-0.476	-∞
8009	-0.002	-0.007	-0.016	-0.029	-0.047	-0.066	-0.102	-0.179	-0.444	-0.576	-0.830	-∞
8010	-0.010	-0.035	-0.091	-0.252	-15.654	-0.333	-0.132	-0.038	0.038	0.054	0.071	0.091
381	0.000	0.000	0.000	0.000	0.000	0.000	0.000	0.000	0.000	0.000	0.000	0.000
442	0.002	0.004	0.005	0.006	0.006	0.006	0.006	0.003	-0.004	-0.007	-0.012	-0.018
Total	1.121	1.285	-0.116	-5.163	-∞	-8.049	-2.523	-1.157	-∞	-6.176	-9.542	-∞

Table VIII. Test of Homogeneity (HOMOG; J. Ott): Reading Disability versus Three Chromosome 15 Markers

H_0: No linkage (α = 0.00, θ = 0.50)
H_1: Linkage with homogeneity (α = 1.00, θ = 0.50)
H_2: Linkage with heterogeneity (α = 0.20, θ = 0.00)

	df	chi-square	p-value
H_2 vs. H_1	1	9.070	0.0013
H_1 vs. H_0	1	0.000	0.5000
H_2 vs. H_0	2	9.070	0.0054

other. This is shown graphically in figure 2, in which the LOD scores for each chromosome at θ = 0.1 are compared for each family, with the families arranged in descending order of the LOD score for chromosome 15.

When the HOMOG analysis was performed with these data from the chromosome 6 markers, α was again estimated to be 20% (table X). The null hypothesis of no linkage was rejected compared to both alternate hypotheses, and the hypothesis of heterogeneity was preferred, but significance levels were not high enough to declare linkage based on these data alone.

In an effort to determine if some of the heterogeneity was contributed by Family 6432, HOMOG was re-run with this family omitted (table XI). The estimate of α increased to 0.85 families linked, and the null hypothesis of no linkage was again rejected, but now the hypothesis of homogeneity could not be rejected when compared to the hypothesis of heterogeneity. Thus, it appears that Family 6432, selected solely on the basis of the linkage results with chromosome 15, contributed to the heterogeneity of linkage seen with chromosome 6, and its omission increased the probability that the remaining families were all linked to chromosome 6. Finally, the significance level reached for linkage with homogeneity would meet Ott's (1985) suggested criteria for acceptance of linkage.

A linkage map showing the results of linkage to chromosome 6 with and without Family 6432 reflects slightly higher total LOD scores, with the highest probability of linkage in the GLO region (figure 3).

Future Studies

Based upon the results of the present study, it can be hypothesized that some families show linkage of reading disability to chromosome 15 but not chromosome 6, and others (a greater proportion) show linkage to chromosome 6 but not 15. In addition to continued studies to increase the number of large families and the number of informative markers for

Table IX. Multipoint Linkage between SRD and Chromosome 6 Markers BF, GLO, and 2C5

Marker					Bf		2C5	GLO				
	0.1	0.2	0.3	0.4	0.5	0.55	0.58	0.60	0.70	0.80	0.90	1.00
Family												
9007	0.048	0.011	-0.178	-0.750	-∞	-1.366	-0.899	-0.694	-0.193	0.003	0.062	0.051
9008	0.129	0.190	0.146	-0.098	-∞	-1.426	-1.487	-1.111	-0.084	0.178	0.222	0.149
9102	0.155	0.487	0.848	1.195	1.519	1.640	1.706	1.749	1.389	0.993	0.570	0.177
381	0.030	0.351	0.748	1.133	1.494	1.474	1.472	1.475	1.109	0.721	0.333	0.045
442	0.061	0.135	0.172	0.060	-∞	-1.141	-1.662	-∞	-0.160	0.102	0.123	0.062
6372	0.071	0.163	0.205	0.132	-0.176	-0.660	-1.371	-∞	-0.160	0.159	0.183	0.086
6375	-0.266	-0.567	-0.980	-1.742	-∞	-5.299	-∞	-2.894	-1.281	-0.763	-0.463	-0.229
6432	**-0.182**	**-0.456**	**-0.949**	**-1.963**	-∞	**-3.991**	**-4.550**	-∞	**-2.776**	**-1.426**	**-0.695**	**-0.249**
6484	0.136	0.154	-0.017	-0.552	-2.248	-4.118	-∞	-2.712	-0.164	0.374	0.434	0.264
6491	0.068	0.245	0.477	0.724	0.964	0.967	0.973	0.978	0.740	0.493	0.257	0.072
6576	-0.078	-0.187	-0.362	-0.690	-1.891	-1.186	-1.392	-∞	-0.605	-0.333	-0.191	-0.090
8001	0.098	0.153	0.125	-0.090	-∞	-2.269	-∞	-∞	-0.483	-0.120	0.008	0.033
8002	-0.001	-0.012	-0.045	-0.114	-0.231	-0.351	-0.415	-0.454	-0.280	-0.128	-0.043	-0.007
8005	-0.002	-0.003	0.004	0.027	0.069	0.104	0.128	0.146	0.067	0.019	-0.001	-0.003
8006	-0.018	-0.076	-0.194	-0.444	-∞	-0.695	-0.531	-0.456	-0.234	-0.116	-0.048	-0.011
8007	0.032	0.056	0.070	0.047	-0.099	-0.425	-∞	-0.543	0.011	0.074	0.062	0.035
8008	-0.017	-0.074	-0.189	-0.429	-1.703	-1.377	-1.475	-1.703	-0.429	-0.189	-0.074	-0.017
8009	0.028	0.463	0.726	0.976	1.204	1.184	1.180	1.180	0.954	0.707	0.448	0.199
8010	-0.004	-0.018	-0.042	-0.078	-0.129	-0.169	-0.197	-0.204	-0.119	-0.063	-0.027	-0.007
Total	0.468	1.015	0.565	-2.656	-∞	-19.104	-∞	-∞	-2.698	0.685	1.160	0.560

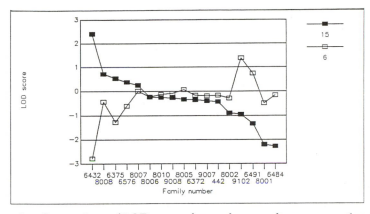

Figure 2. Comparison of LOD scores for markers on chromosomes 6 and 15. The families are listed along the x-axis in descending order of their LOD scores for chromosome 15 heteromorphisms at 10% recombination. These scores are indicated by the closed circles. The LOD scores for the chromosome 6 markers at 10% recombination for each family are shown by the open squares.

these two regions, two other approaches to gene localization will be utilized, namely the affected sib-pair method (Blackwelder and Elston 1985) and the method of interval mapping for quantitative trait loci (Lander and Botstein 1989).

The sib-pair method is based on the assumption that, if a major gene for a trait is tightly linked to a marker gene, a pair of sibs who are both affected with the trait will also tend to be concordant for the same linked allele. A significant discrepancy from random assortment of the trait and the marker allele can be taken as evidence for linkage. This is not as powerful as the family study method, and is generally used as a screen for candidate loci for more intensive family studies, but it also has some advantages over the family study method that are particularly appropriate for the study of reading disability. The primary advantages are that it can be used to test for a locus conferring a non-Mendelian susceptibility for a trait and that assumptions about the

Table X. Test of Homogeneity (HOMOG; J. Ott): Reading Disability versus Chromosome 6 Markers

H_0: No linkage ($\alpha = 0.00$, $\theta = 0.50$)
H_1: Linkage with homogeneity ($\alpha = 1.00$, $\theta = 0.30$)
H_2: Linkage with heterogeneity ($\alpha = 0.20$, $\theta = 0.00$)

	df	chi-square	p-value
H_2 vs. H_1	1	2.947	0.0430
H_1 vs. H_0	1	5.342	0.0104
H_2 vs. H_0	2	8.289	0.0079

Table XI.   Test of Homogeneity (HOMOG; J. Ott): Reading Disability versus
Chromosome 6 Markers, Family 6432 Omitted

H_0: No linkage ($\alpha = 0.00$, $\theta = 0.50$)
H_1: Linkage with homogeneity ($\alpha = 1.00$, $\theta = 0.20$)
H_2: Linkage with heterogeneity ($\alpha = 0.85$, $\theta = 0.20$)

	df	chi-square	p-value
H_2 vs. H_1	1	0.364	0.2731
H_1 vs. H_0	1	9.722	0.0009
H_2 vs. H_0	2	10.086	0.0032

mode of inheritance or penetrance of the trait do not need to be made. In addition, other family members do not need to be diagnosed, which alleviates the problem of compensation. However, the markers must be highly polymorphic so that alleles that are shared can be assumed to be identical by descent. Preliminary computations with informative sib pairs in our families show that neither chromosome 15 heteromorphisms nor GLO types show significant sharing; however, only 9 sibships (25 sib pairs) could be unambiguously scored for chromosome 15, and only 14 sibships (37 pairs) could be scored for number of shared GLO alleles (0–1 versus 1–2). Clearly, these single loci are not polymorphic enough for this analysis, and multiple loci must be used.

The methods for searching for quantitative trait loci (Lander and Botstein 1989) will also be very useful in identifying chromosomal regions for further analysis. Since multiple chromosomal regions can be

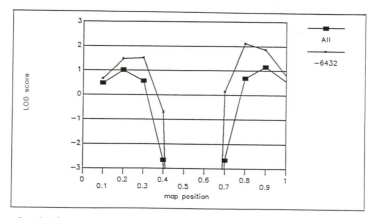

Figure 3.   Linkage map of chromosome 6 with SRD with and without Family 6432. The x-axis represents the relative genetic position of the markers (in recombination units) along the long arm of the chromosome. The multipoint LOD scores for the total population studied are shown by the closed circles. As indicated by the open boxes, the LOD scores for chromosome 6 markers increase when the scores from Family 6432 are subtracted from the total.

considered simultaneously, it may be possible to begin to assess the extent to which reading deficits are due to individual quantitative trait loci.

CONCLUDING REMARKS

During the past five years, several important results have been obtained by co-investigators associated with the Colorado Reading Project. Within the Twin/Family Study component, a new multiple regression analysis of twin data has been developed that provides compelling evidence for a genetic etiology of reading disability. In addition to being statistically powerful, this methodology is highly flexible and is presently being used by Colorado Reading Project investigators to test various hypotheses that are relevant to important issues in the field of learning disabilities. For example, we are currently employing the multiple regression analysis of twin data to validate alternative typologies and evaluate the assumption of specificity (Foorman 1989; Stanovich 1986).

Within the Reading and Language Processes component, investigators have found that disabled readers have phonological coding skills that are well below the levels expected on the basis of their word recognition skills, whereas their performance on an orthographic task is slightly better than expected. Moreover, employing a bivariate form of the multiple regression analysis of twin data, evidence has been obtained to indicate that the correlation between phonological coding and word recognition is largely due to heritable influences, whereas the relationship between orthographic coding and word recognition is due primarily to environmental influences.

Within the Epidemiology of Immunological Differences component, no association has been found between reading disability and prevalence of immune disorders. However, comparisons of MZ and DZ concordance rates suggested the possible validity of a genetic subtype of reading disability with atopic disorders, a result which is convergent with the preliminary evidence for linkage between reading disability and chromosome 6 found in the Linkage Analysis component.

Results obtained by co-investigators within the Linkage Analysis component strongly suggest that reading disability is etiologically heterogeneous. For example, the co-investigators have found that about 20% of families with apparent autosomal dominant transmission for reading disability manifest linkage to chromosome 15, but not to chromosome 6. Some evidence for linkage to chromosome 6, but not to 15, was obtained from data on other families. The co-investigators are currently increasing their sample size and the number of informative markers on chromosomes 15 and 6, and are beginning to employ the method of interval mapping to search for quantitative trait loci that may influence reading disability.

In addition to these within-component analyses, several cross-component analyses are also currently in progress. For example, using state-of-the-art segregation analysis computer programs, currently we are conducting a genetic analysis of data from over 400 families that have been ascertained within the various components. Another example is a linkage analysis of data from fraternal twins in which our multiple regression analyses of twin data will be used to assess the extent to which the reading performance deficit of probands is due to quantitative trait loci. In this manner, the methods of quantitative genetics, developmental psychology, clinical psychology, and medical genetics are being combined to obtain a more complete understanding of the etiology of reading disability.

REFERENCES

Bakwin, H. 1973. Reading disability in twins. *Developmental Medicine and Child Neurology* 15:184–87.

Blackwelder, W. C., and Elston, R. C. 1985. A comparison of sib-pair linkage tests for disease susceptibility loci. *Genetic Epidemiology* 2:85–97.

Bryant, P. E., and Goswami, U. C. 1986. Strengths and weaknesses of the reading level design: A comment on Backman, Mamen, and Ferguson. *Psychological Bulletin* 100:101–103.

Cohen, J. 1977. *Statistical Power Analysis for the Behavioral Sciences.* New York: Academic Press.

Cohen, J., and Cohen, P. 1975. *Applied Multiple Regression/Correlation Analysis for the Behavioral Sciences.* Hillsdale, NJ: Lawrence Erlbaum Associates.

Conners, F., and Olson, R. (in press). Reading comprehension in dyslexic and normal readers: A component skills analysis. In *Comprehension Processes in Reading,* eds. D. A. Balota, G. B. Flores d'Arcais, and K. Rayner. Hillsdale, NJ: Lawrence Erlbaum Associates.

Decker, S. N., and Vandenberg, S. G. 1985. Colorado twin study of reading disability. In *Biobehavioral Measures of Dyslexia,* eds. D. B. Gray and J. F. Kavanagh. Parkton, MD: York Press.

DeFries, J. C. 1985. Colorado reading project. In *Biobehavioral Measures of Dyslexia,* eds. D. B. Gray and J. F. Kavanagh. Parkton, MD: York Press.

DeFries, J. C., and Fulker, D. W. 1985. Multiple regression analysis of twin data. *Behavior Genetics* 15:467–73.

DeFries, J. C., and Fulker, D. W. 1988. Multiple regression analysis of twin data: Etiology of deviant scores versus individual differences. *Acta Geneticae Medicae et Gemellologiae: Twin Research* 37:205–16.

DeFries, J. C., and Gillis, J. J. (in press). Etiology of reading deficits in learning disabilities: Quantitative genetic analysis. In *Advances in the Neuropsychology of Learning Disabilities: Issues, Methods and Practice,* eds. J. E. Obrzut and G. W. Hynd. Orlando, FL: Academic Press.

Dunn, L. M., and Markwardt, F. C. 1970. *Examiner's Manual: Peabody Individual Achievement Test.* Circle Pines, MN: American Guidance Service.

Finucci, J. M. 1978. Genetic considerations in dyslexia. In *Progress in Learning Disabilities*, Vol. IV, ed. H. R. Myklebust. New York: Grune and Stratton.

Finucci, J. M., Guthrie, J. T., Childs, A. L., Abbey, H., and Childs, B. 1976. The genetics of specific reading disability. *Annals of Human Genetics* (London) 40: 1–23.

Foorman, B. R. 1989. What's specific about specific reading disability: An introduction to the special series. *Journal of Learning Disabilities* 22:332–33.

Geschwind, N., and Behan, P. O. 1982. Left-handedness: Association with immune disease, migraine, and developmental learning disorder. *Proceedings of the National Academy of Sciences* 79:5097–5100.

Geschwind, N., and Behan, P. O. 1984. Laterality, hormones, and immunity. In *Cerebral Dominance: The Biological Foundations*, eds. N. Geschwind and A. Galaburda. Cambridge, MA: Harvard University Press.

Geschwind, N., and Galaburda, A. M. 1985. Cerebral lateralization: Biological mechanisms, associations, and pathology: II. A hypothesis and a program for research. *Archives of Neurology* 42:521–52.

Gilger, J. W., Pennington, B. F., and DeFries, J. C. in review. Using twin data to assess the etiology of comorbid disorders.

Gray, D. B., and Kavanagh, J. F. (eds.). 1985. *Biobehavioral Measures of Dyslexia.* Parkton, MD: York Press.

Hallgren, B. 1950. Specific dyslexia ("congenital word-blindness"): A clinical and genetic study. *Acta Psychiatrica et Neurologica Scandinavia*, Suppl. 65.

Haseman, J. K., and Elston, R. C. 1972. The investigation of linkage between a quantitative trait and a marker locus. *Behavior Genetics* 2:3–19.

Kaufman, A. S. 1975. Factor analysis of the WISC-R at 11 age levels between 6½ and 16½ years. *Journal of Consulting and Clinical Psychology* 43:135–47.

LaBuda, M. C., DeFries, J. C., and Pennington, B. F. 1990. Reading disability: A model for the genetic analysis of complex behavioral disorders. *Journal of Counseling and Development* 68:645–51.

Lander, E. S., and Botstein, D. 1986. Strategies for studying heterogeneous genetic traits in humans by using a linkage map of restriction fragment length polymorphisms. *Proceedings of the National Academy of Sciences* 83:7353–7357.

Lander, E. S., and Botstein, D. 1989. Mapping Mendelian factors underlying quantitative traits using RFLP linkage maps. *Genetics* 121:185–99.

Lathrop, G. M., Lalouel, J. M., Julier, C., and Ott, J. 1985. Multilocus linkage analysis in humans: Detection of linkage and estimation of recombination. *American Journal of Human Genetics* 37:482–98.

Lewitter, F. I., DeFries, J. C., and Elston, R. C. 1980. Genetic models of reading disability. *Behavior Genetics* 10:9–30.

Lykken, D. T., Tellegen, A., and DeRubeis, R. 1978. Volunteer bias in twin research: The rule of two-thirds. *Social Biology* 25:1–9.

Morton, N. E. 1955. Sequential tests for the detection of linkage. *American Journal of Human Genetics* 7:277–318.

Morton, N. E. 1956. The detection and estimation of linkage between the genes for elliptocytosis and the Rh blood type. *American Journal of Human Genetics* 19:23–24.

Nichols, R. C., and Bilbro, W. C. 1966. The diagnosis of twin zygosity. *Acta Genetica* 16:265–75.

Olson, R. K. 1985. Disabled reading processes and cognitive profiles. In *Biobehavioral Measures of Dyslexia*, eds. D. B. Gray and J. F. Kavanagh. Parkton, MD: York Press.

Olson, R. K., Kliegl, R., Davidson, B. J., and Foltz, G. 1985. Individual and developmental differences in reading disability. In *Reading Research: Ad-*

vances in Theory and Practice, Vol. 4, eds. G. E. MacKinnon and T. G. Waller. New York: Academic Press.

Olson, R. K., Rack, J. P., Conners, F. A., DeFries, J. C., and Fulker, D. W. (in press-a). Genetic etiology of individual differences in reading disability. In *Subtypes of Learning Disability,* eds. L. V. Feagans, E. J. Shart, and L. J. Meltzer. Hillsdale, NJ: Lawrence Erlbaum Associates.

Olson, R. K., Wise, B., Conners, F. A., and Rack, J. P. (in press-b). Organization, heritability, and remediation of component word recognition and language skills in disabled readers. In *Reading and Its Development: Component Skills Approaches,* eds. T. H. Carr and B. A. Levy. New York: Academic Press.

Olson, R. K., Wise, B., Conners, F., Rack, J., and Fulker, D. 1989. Specific deficits in component reading and language skills: Genetic and environmental influences. *Journal of Learning Disabilities* 22:339–48.

Ott, J. 1985. *Analysis of Human Genetic Linkage.* Baltimore: The Johns Hopkins University Press.

Pennington, B. F., Smith, S. D., Kimberling, W. J., Green, P., and Haith, M. M. 1987. Left-handedness and immune disorders in familial dyslexics: A test of Geschwind's hypothesis. *Archives of Neurology* 44:634–39.

Pennington, B. F., Smith, S. D., McCabe, L. L., Kimberling, W. J., and Lubs, H. A. 1984. Developmental continuities and discontinuities in a form of familial dyslexia. In *Continuities and Discontinuities in Development,* eds. R. Emde and R. Harman. New York: Plenum.

Plomin, R., DeFries, J. C., and McClearn, G. E. 1990. *Behavioral Genetics: A Primer.* San Francisco: W. H. Freeman.

Rack, J. P., and Olson, R. K. 1989. Sources of variance in the phonological deficit in developmental dyslexia. Paper presented at the meeting of the Rodin Remediation Society, September 1989, Bangor, Wales.

Rack, J. P., Snowling, M. J., and Olson, R. K. (submitted). The nonword reading deficit in developmental dyslexia: A review.

Rutter, M., and Yule, W. 1975. The concept of specific reading retardation. *Journal of Child Psychology and Psychiatry* 16:181–97.

Shucard, D. W., Cummins, K. R., Gay, E., Lairsmith, J., and Welanko, P. 1985. Electrophysiological studies of reading-disabled children: In search of subtypes. In *Biobehavioral Measures of Dyslexia,* eds. D. B. Gray and J. F. Kavanagh. Parkton, MD: York Press.

Smith, S. D., Kimberling, W. J., Pennington, B. F., and Lubs, H. A. 1983. Specific reading disability: Identification of an inherited form through linkage analysis. *Science* 219:1345–1347.

Snowling, M. J. 1980. The development of grapheme-phoneme correspondence in normal and dyslexic readers. *Journal of Experimental Child Psychology* 29:294–305.

Stanovich, K. E. 1986. Cognitive processes and the reading problems of learning-disabled children: Evaluating the assumption of specificity. In *Psychological and Educational Perspectives on Learning Disabilities,* eds. J. K. Torgesen and B. Y. L. Wong. Orlando, FL: Academic Press.

Stanovich, K. E. 1989. Has the LD field lost its intelligence? *Journal of Learning Disabilities* 22:487–92.

Stanovich, K. E., and West, R. F. 1989. Exposure to print and orthographic processing. *Reading Research Quarterly* 24:402–433.

Stevenson, J., Graham, P., Fredman, G., and McLoughlin, V. 1987. A twin study of genetic influences on reading and spelling ability and disability. *Journal of Child Psychology and Psychiatry* 28:229–47.

Treiman, R., and Hirsh-Pasek, K. 1985. Are there qualitative differences in reading behavior between dyslexic and normal readers? *Memory and Cognition* 13:357–64.

Van Orden, G. C. 1987. A ROWS is a ROSE: Spelling, sound and reading. *Memory and Cognition* 15:181–98.

Vogel, S. A. 1990. Gender differences in intelligence, language, visual-motor abilities, and academic achievement in students with learning disabilities: A review of the literature. *Journal of Learning Disabilities* 23:44–52.

Wadsworth, S. J., Gillis, J. J., and DeFries, J. C. 1990. Genetic etiology of reading disability as a function of age. *Behavior Genetics* 20.

Wechsler, D. 1974. *Examiner's Manual: Wechsler Intelligence Scale for Children–Revised*. New York: The Psychological Corporation.

Wechsler, D. 1981. *Examiner's Manual: Wechsler Adult Intelligence Scale–Revised*. New York: The Psychological Corporation.

Wong, B. Y. L. 1986. Problems and issues in the definition of learning disabilities. In *Psychological and Educational Perspectives on Learning Disabilities*, eds. J. K. Torgesen and B. Y. L. Wong. Orlando, FL: Academic Press.

Zerbin-Rüdin, E. 1967. Kongenitale Wortblindheit oder spezifische dyslixie (Congenital Word-Blindness). *Bulletin of The Orton Society* 17:47–56.

Chapter • **4**

Dyslexia Subtypes
Genetics, Behavior, and Brain Imaging

Herbert A. Lubs, Ranjan Duara,
Bonnie Levin, Bonnie Jallad,
Marie-Louise Lubs, Mark Rabin,
Alex Kushch, and Karen Gross-Glenn

The first purpose of the study is to define the chromosomal location of the several genes that produce autosomal dominantly inherited dyslexia. The second purpose is to define the effects that each of these different genes produces on the form and function of the brains of people with these variant genes, not only in respect to reading and writing, but on all aspects of brain function that we can study. If similar clinical problems are inherited in a polygenic, autosomal recessive, and x-linked fashion, then, by definition, multiple disorders and genes are involved. Moreover, if information from families with each of those different disorders is pooled, it is very difficult to interpret the resulting data. In this study, therefore, we chose to include only three-generation families with an autosomal dominant (AD) mode of inheritance in order to simplify the data analysis. This is probably the most frequent form of inheritance of dyslexia. Equal numbers of males and females are affected and half of offspring from a parent who has the gene are also affected. Even with the limitation to families showing AD inheritance, it is still likely that multiple genes are in-

This work was supported by a grant from NICHD (#PO1-HD21885) to Herbert A. Lubs. We thank C. Brown for assistance in manuscript preparation.

volved in the genesis of dyslexia and that subtle differences will be found between different AD genetic types.

This is a very different study from others presented in this volume and it is also a different study from any that have been carried out previously. Once we have identified the several genes for dyslexia, we can then utilize the data from the wide variety of test procedures used in the study to define the effects of the presumed several genes. We are not starting with a definition based upon a laboratory or behavioral test. Rather, we start with a gene and then define its clinical expression or phenotypes. It is a biologic approach to the definition of the various subtypes of dyslexia.

Background of the Present Study

Genetics is the study of individual variation. Each person has, roughly, a hundred thousand functional genes. This information is encoded in our DNA by more than three billion base pairs. A project to map this genome is in the planning stage now, and will be the largest biological study that has ever been done. The data generated from this study will actually exceed the capacity of the largest computers that are now used. Within ten years, significant data will come from it and in twenty perhaps, it will be completed. Ultimately, it will help this study immensely by providing new markers and new information about our genome.

The present study will require ten years to complete. It is an extremely complex undertaking for both investigators and the dedicated family members who participate in all aspects of the project. It requires over 20 hours of testing for each family member, over 4 or 5 days. Approximately 350 variables of all types are recorded, at least on those individuals who participate in all aspects of the study. If we are successful, our view of dyslexia will be quite changed.

The predecessor to this study began about 15 years ago, when Shelley Smith came to do her thesis in Denver with one of us (HL). As a clinical geneticist interested in the application of genetics to common problems, I suggested a study of a little-investigated disorder—namely dominantly inherited dyslexia. The broad goal of this first study was to provide additional support for the idea that there was a group of families with dyslexia due to autosomal dominant inheritance. Since we were starting with three-generation families with apparent autosomal dominant inheritance, such a study might be viewed as a self-fulfilling prophecy. We decided, in addition, to do a linkage study. The nature of the linkage study, which determines the frequency with which two genes are inherited together through a large family, has as its basis for accepting a linkage the fact that the results are not likely due to chance. The likelihood of flipping a coin and having it come up heads ten times in a row is $1/2^{10}$ or $1/1024$. That is essentially the same likelihood that two genes will be inherited together in 10 transmissions through a family by chance. The first step in detecting a linkage is to recognize co-transmission of genes that occurs a 1000 times more likely than chance alone. Thus there are few false positive results. The second step is to repeat the study to confirm the findings. Since we were unlikely to find a false positive result, we felt a positive study would confirm that there was at least one autosomal dominant gene leading to dyslexia. This was the basis of the initial study that Drs. Smith, Kimberling, and I undertook. Dr. Pennington later also became involved in extending the family data.

To understand linkage studies fully, however, the behavior of chromosomes in meiosis must be understood. Not only do homologous chromosomes pair (No. 1 with No. 2, etc.), but an average of two crossovers, or exchanges, occur in each of the 23 pairs of chromosomes. These recombinations occur randomly throughout each chromosome and result in greater biologic mixing; they also provide geneticists with a means of doing detailed linkage studies using normal variations in the genetic code, called restriction fragment length polymorphisms (or RFLPs). The likelihood with which any two variant genes will be inherited together depends on how close they are on the same chromosome. If they are extremely close, they will nearly always be transmitted together to one child, and another child of the same parents will almost always get both normal genes. If two genes are far apart on the chromosome or on different chromosomes, the inheritance of the two genes will be totally random. Thus, the closer together the genes are, the more likely we will be to find such linkage. The ideal study would utilize a series of markers equally distributed through the 23 chromosomes: about 200 RFLPs would yield a good probability of detecting a linkage to a disease gene. That is too expensive to do routinely, so we must take another approach, namely to pursue specific clues about possible localizations or linkages.

A few additional terms must be defined. The frequency of recombination is indicated by the symbol *theta* (θ); a 1% recombination rate was defined in classical genetics as one centimorgan. In molecular terms, one centimorgan, or a 1% recombination frequency, is equivalent to about one million base pairs. This is roughly the size of our largest known disease gene, the Duchenne muscular dystrophy gene. Results of linkage studies are given in terms of the Log of Odds of linkage, or the so-called LOD score. A LOD score of $+3$, for example, indicates that the odds are a thousand to one ($10^3/1$) in favor of linkage over a random occurrence of the same findings. A low score, less than -2.0 ($1/10^2$) indicates that the odds are 100/1 against linkage. These are the usual levels for accepting or rejecting a linkage between two genes. Since the odds are expressed as base 10 logarithmic data, a score can be accumulated over a period of time from a number of families by summing these LOD scores. When Dr. Smith began the initial study in the early 1970s the distribution of the markers was limited. Many were genes for blood groups and are, including the Rh locus, now known to be on chromosome 1. There are five chromosomes—13, 14, 15, 21, and 22—with small, variable short arms; these variations were used as "chromosomal markers." Similarly, variations in protein were also used as markers in linkage studies. In the study reported by Smith et al. (1983), there were no markers on chromosomes 4 or 5 for example, and we could not have detected a linkage on either chromosome. Overall, only about 20% of the genome was studied. Current studies, including the more recent reports of Smith et al. (1990a, 1990b) and the present study are slightly more inclusive but still leave many gaps in the genome due to a lack of useful, inexpensive markers to detect.

The families included in this study had a number of family members with major problems in reading and spelling. Each person's intelligence was normal and no reason for the reading difficulty was known. This study group, however, was significantly different from prior study groups because now we required a three-generation family history with the same problem. These results were published (Smith et al. 1983) when the LOD score exceeded 3.0 between dyslexia and short arm variations on chromosome 15. These studies have continued and have been summarized (Smith et al. 1990b). The results of the current linkage analysis of dyslexia and chromosome 15 heteromorphisms is shown in table I (reprinted from Smith et al. 1990b). Fourteen new families were added and five of the eight families published in 1983 were extended.

Both inspection of the data in table I and a formal analysis for genetic heterogeneity lead to the conclusion that more than one locus for dyslexia exists (Smith et al. 1990a, 1990b). Family 432, which contributed most of the initial information leading to a total LOD score greater than 3.0 in the eight initial study families, was the subject of further study and now yielded an LOD score of 2.961. No crossovers were observed ($\theta = 0$) and it is quite likely that a gene exists near the centromere of 15 that results in a phenotype with dyslexia. Overall, 18% of the 20 families were found to fit the hypothesis of linkage to a gene on 15. Thus, both further studies of chromosome 15 using new markers adjacent to the centromere as well as a continued search for loci on other chromosomes is appropriate. The family data continued to be consistent with an autosomal dominant mode (AD) of inheritance both in the newly studied families and the extended studies of the original families. The latter observation, of course, is particularly important evi-

Table I.   Linkage between SRD and Chromosome 15 Heteromorphisms

Family	Recombination Fraction				
	0.00	0.10	0.20	0.30	0.40
9007	$-\infty$	-0.384	-0.047	0.032	0.020
9008	$-\infty$	-0.264	-0.109	-0.049	-0.015
9102	$-\infty$	-0.957	-0.426	-0.168	-0.040
6372	$-\infty$	-0.350	0.614	0.276	0.201
6375	0.628	0.535	0.370	0.191	0.051
6432	2.907	2.401	1.877	1.323	0.712
6484	$-\infty$	-2.279	-0.750	-0.141	0.060
6491	$-\infty$	-1.332	-0.582	-0.228	-0.054
6576	0.523	0.334	0.180	0.071	0.015
8001	$-\infty$	-2.201	-1.114	-0.553	-0.215
8002	$-\infty$	-0.888	-0.297	-0.084	-0.014
8005	-1.703	-0.335	-0.122	-0.038	-0.006
8006	$-\infty$	0.159	0.232	0.182	0.093
8007	0.301	0.255	0.204	0.146	0.079
8008	0.903	0.725	0.541	0.356	0.175
8010	$-\infty$	-0.252	-0.092	-0.036	-0.010
6371	0.602	0.465	0.318	0.170	0.049
1000	0.292	0.208	0.129	0.062	0.016
1001	$-\infty$	-0.229	-0.060	-0.011	-0.001
1002	0.292	0.208	0.129	0.062	0.016
Total	$-\infty$	-4.181	0.995	1.563	1.132

LOD scores are given for each family at 5 values of θ; 0.00, 0.10, 0.20, 0.30, and 0.40. The symbol minus infinity ($-\infty$) at $\theta = 0.00$ indicates that a crossover event has taken place. By convention, a LOD score less than or equal to -2.0 excludes linkage at that value of θ, and a LOD score of at least 3.0 is evidence of linkage. SRD is standard reading disability.

(Taken from Smith, Pennington, Kimberling, and Ing 1990)

dence in favor of the hypothesis of AD inheritance and against multi-factorial or a non-genetic origin of the newly ascertained cases.

THE PRESENT STUDY

Criteria for Entry into the Study

Families with a three-generation history of relatively pure dyslexia are candidates for admission into the study. Generally, at least ten potentially informative matings are required for each family. As in prior studies, dyslexia is initially defined as a significant difficulty in reading and spelling in persons with no medical or neurological disorders, a normal intelligence, and adequate educational opportunity. Only primary English speaking families are considered. A questionnaire relating to medical, educational, and behavioral history is given to each person (Lubs et al. in press). The majority of family members reside in south Florida so that many of the special studies, which require special equipment, can be carried out. An IQ test and a variety of reading, vision, speech, and neuropsychological studies are administered to as many affected and normal family members as possible. Magnetic resonance imaging (MRI) and positron-emission tomography (PET) studies are carried out in a smaller number of family members. In figure 1 each person is given a unique number (shown above the circles or squares in the pedigrees).

The diagnostic screening battery includes a standard intelligence test and tests for reading and spelling skills. These are divided into four classes of subtests, as shown in figure 1: those that measure oral reading, comprehension, decoding, or spelling. Criteria for diagnosis of dyslexia changes with the age or grade of the child. In the first year of school, a score only half a standard deviation below their expected score (based on IQ) is required in at least one of the four categories (see figure 1). This increases to one standard deviation for the age group 9–14 years, on two of the four categories, and to 1.5 standard deviations on two of the four categories for those age 15 or over. The Nonsense Passages, initially described by Finucci et al. (1976) have been particularly helpful. This test removes guessing as an effective strategy. Dyslexics generally have shown either a need for increased time to read the passages correctly or an increased number of errors (Gross-Glenn et al. 1985, 1990).

Results of Family Studies

To date, of 14 families initially entered in the study, 10 have proven appropriate and sufficiently motivated to participate. Sufficient data to warrant presentation at this time are available from five families. Pedigrees of three families are shown in figure 2, as are the explanations for the pedigree symbols. Pedigrees of the remaining two families are presented in the section on neuropsychological studies. Two individuals (Families 3015-253 and 258) were dyslexic by history but psychometric test results did not meet the criteria for a diagnosis of dyslexia. Rarely, a person such as 3015-237 will be negative by history and by testing but will transmit the presumed gene. Such an individual represents an example of decreased penetrance. This occurred in only one individual of 53 who were clearly affected, had a history of dyslexia, or clearly transmitted the gene. Such decreased penetrance occurs frequently with dominant inheritance of all types and a penetrance rate of about 90% should not be considered in any way unusual or to weaken

Diagnostic Reading/Spelling Battery
and
Criteria for Diagnosis of Dyslexia

1. Spelling   Wide-Range Achievement Test-Revised:
Spelling subtest

2. Oral Reading   Gray-Oral Reading Test-Revised
Woodcock-Johnson Psycho-Educational Battery
Letter-Word Identification subtest

3. Comprehension   Woodcock-Johnson Psycho-Educational Battery
Passage Comprehension subtest

4. Decoding   Woodcock-Johnson Psycho-Educational Battery
Word-Attack Scale subtest
Nonsense Passages (ages 16+)

****

IQ Discrepancy (in comparison to IQ score)	Grade	Age-graded cutoffs
$\geq$ 0.5 standard deviation on 1 out of 4 reading and spelling tests	< 3	$\leq$ 8 years
$\geq$ 1.0 standard deviation on 2 out of 4 reading and spelling tests	3 - 8	9 - 14 years
$\geq$ 1.5 standard deviations on 2 out of 4 reading and spelling tests	> 8	$\geq$ 15 years

Figure 1. Age-graded cutoffs.

the concept of a single gene of dyslexia. Because of the large three-generation families and the transmission to an equal number of offspring of both sexes of the normal and dyslexic genes, the current families provide strong additional support for AD inheritance in a significant portion of cases of dyslexia. The exact proportion of cases of similarly "pure" dyslexia (having problems primarily with reading and spelling) remains unknown, but probably represents a significant proportion of all cases.

It is often stated that there is a 3:1 or 4:1 ratio of diagnosed males to females with dyslexia. Three of the four people who showed no currently detectable effects of the gene(s) but transmitted it in these five

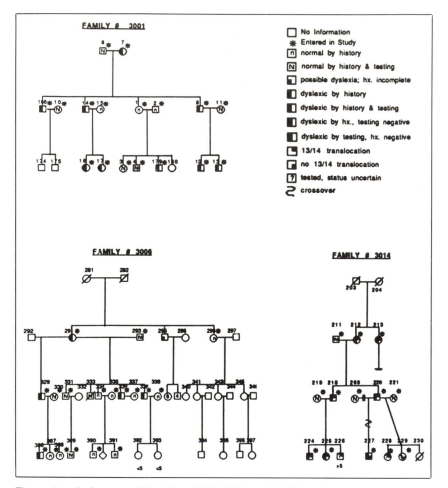

Figure 2.   Pedigrees of families, 3001, 3006, and 3014.

pedigrees were females. We have suspected for some time that in general the females in the families are less severely affected. Our current data support this concept. The sex ratio is equal within these families and those of Smith et al. (1983). It appears, therefore, that the higher rate of diagnosis in males results from a greater severity in males, i.e., a threshold effect; perhaps, also, the more active behavior of males in classrooms results in more frequent attention and diagnosis. We are, of course, examining the results of the test battery carefully to determine whether individuals #237 and #241, and others with similar histories and test results, show any evidence of being unusual or abnormal. This approach may lead to a test that would detect all individuals with a gene for dyslexia and would greatly simplify the study of dyslexia.

Family #3015 is an example of an excellent family for the study.

There are 23 potentially informative matings. This family alone, if there were no crossovers, could give significant evidence for a linkage. The chance of co-inheritance of dyslexia and a marker without linkage is only $1/2^{23}$.

We are looking for possible linkages with conventional approaches to avoid carrying out the approximately 200 DNA tests on every person and every family that are otherwise required. One study family (3014) has a Robertsonian translocation with a centrometric fusion of chromosomes 13 and 14, and dyslexia. Individuals with this translocation are perfectly normal although they have only 45 chromosomes. Initially it was reported that everyone with this translocation also had dyslexia, and they were included in our study. With more detailed studies, only 6 of the 7 family members have both the translocation and dyslexia (see Family 3014, figure 2). The two children (228 and 229) still are being evaluated for dyslexia. The "wiggle" above patient 227 indicates there is a clear separation of the translocation and dyslexia, and would be an example of a crossover if the gene were close to the centromere. This family, at least, represents a possible clue that there might be another gene for dyslexia on chromosome 13 or 14.

The second approach to the detection of possible linkage involves the use of the "classical" blood group and protein markers. These are relatively inexpensive and can be run on each family. As in the initial study 15 years ago with these markers, and also by the current slightly larger batteries, less than 25% of the genome is screened. The distribution and frequency of these and other markers are shown in figure 3 and table II.

Our initial laboratory effort, using normal DNA variants (RFLPs), has been directed at developing appropriately located and informative probes in the region of the long arm of chromosome 15 (15q), so that the reports of Smith et al. (1983, 1990a, 1990b) can be confirmed. Because there were few available informative probes in this region, much of the preliminary work has involved probe development. Details of these studies have been given elsewhere (Lubs et al. 1990). Cell lines are established on all family members who participate in the linkage study. To date, no data suggestive of linkage to chromosome 15 have been found in our families. The two probes reported by Smith (1990a, 1990b) were located quite distally on 15q and the absence of evidence for significant linkage was, therefore, to be expected. Similarly, the small negative study of five two-generation Danish families (Bisgaard et al. 1987), using chromosomal heteromorphisms, does not negate the findings in Family 432 and is difficult to interpret since diagnosis was by history alone. Restudy of Family 432 will be critical in confirming or refuting the chromosome 15 linkage, and in determining the direction of linkage studies in the future.

Three additional clues have emerged from the studies with classi-

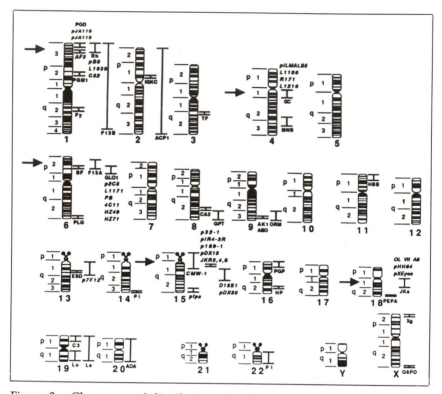

Figure 3. Chromosomal distribution of polymorphic protein markers (solid text) and DNA markers (outline text) used in the study of Smith et al. 1983 and the current University of Miami linkage studies. Subchromosomal localization of respective probes is indicated. The DNA markers are listed in table III.

cal markers. In two of our families (3001, 3015) there were positive LOD scores with GLO (glyoxylase), a marker for a locus on 6p (a total LOD score of 1.3, with no crossovers). Since Smith et al. (personal communication) also have noted slightly positive LOD scores with GLO, this appears to be the most interesting new possible linkage. These and other positive LOD scores are summarized in table III and figure 4. Both the Rh blood group (1p) and GC (4q) have slightly positive LOD scores in two families. We are currently pursuing these clues using RFLPs in these regions.

In summary, there are several possible, but no confirmed linkages. Large numbers of families and several years of study will be required to detect and confirm the linkage with the several (presumed) genes leading to AD inherited dyslexia.

Immunologic Studies. We are attempting to characterize all possible pertinent aspects of individuals with genetic dyslexia. For this

Table II.   Polymorphic Protein Markers

System	Symbol	Chromosome Locus	No. Alleles
α 1-Antitrypsin	PI	14q32.1	5
ABO Blood Group+	ABO	9q34.1-q34.2	4
Acid Phosphatase+	ACP1	2	2
Adenosine Deaminase+	ADA	20	2
Adenylate kinase	AK1	9q34.1-q34.2	2
Carbonic Anhydrase*	CA2	9q22	2
Coagulation Factor 13A	F13A	6p24-p21.3	3
Coagulation Factor 13B	F13B	1	3
Complement (Third Component)	C3	1p13.3-p13.2	2
Complement (Fourth Component)	C4	6p21.3	28
Duffy Blood Group+	FY1	q22-q23	3
Esterase D+	ESD	13q14.1-q14.2	2
Glucose-6-Phosphaste Dehydrogenase*+	G6PD	Xq28	3
Glutamic Pyruvic Transaminase	GPT	8q23-qter	2
Glyoxylase	GLO1	6p21.3-p21.1	3
Group Specific Component+	GC	4q12-q13	2
Haptoglobin+	HP	16q22	2
Hemoglobin*	HBB	11p15.5	2
Immunoglobulin Gm+	IGHG	14q32,3	3
Immunoglobulin Km	IGKC	2p12	2
Kidd Blood Group+	Jk	18q11-q12	2
Lewis Blood Group	Le	19	2
Lutheran Blood Group	Lu	19q12-q13	2
MNS Blood Group+	MNS	4q28-q31	4
Orosomucoid	ORM	9q31-qter	2
P Blood Group	P1	22q11.2-qter	2
Peptidase A*	PEPA	18q23	3
Phosphoglucomutase+	PGM1	1p22.1	4
Phosphogluconate Dehydrogenase	PGD	1p36.2-p36.13	2
Phosphoglycolate Phosphatase	PGP	16p13	3
Plasminogen	PLG	6q26-q27	3
Properdin Factor B	BF	6p21.3	2
Rhesus Blood Group+	Rh	1p36.2-p34	5
Transferrin+	TF	3q21	3
Xg Blood Group	Xg	Xp22.3	2

  *Blacks only
  +Smith et al. 1983a

reason, we are pursuing the suggestion of Geschwind and Galaburda (1985) that there might be a relationship between immunologic abnormalities, left-handedness, and dyslexia. There has, however, not been an increased frequency of non-righthandedness in our study sample

Table III.   Maximal LOD Scores for Polymorphic Markers in Miami Families (θ = 0.0)

Chromosome	Marker	3001	3006	Family 3014	3015	3017
1p36.2-p36.13	PGD	0.00	0.00	0.003	$-\infty$	0.00
1p36.2-p34	Rh	$-\infty$	$-\infty$	0.98	$-\infty$	0.54
1p22.1	PGM1	$-\infty$	0.00	0.27	$-\infty$	0.00
1p13.3-p13.2	C3	0.00	-0.02	$-\infty$	$-\infty$	0.055
1q22-q23	Fy	0.00	0.29	0.18	0.10	$-\infty$
1	F13B	0.00	0.00	0.057	0.08	0.00
2	ACP1	0.00	0.00	0.09	$-\infty$	0.00
3q21	TF	0.00	0.00	0.002	0.0003	0.002
4q12-q13	GC	$-\infty$	0.90	0.06	$-\infty$	0.45
4q28-q31	MNS	$-\infty$	$-\infty$	$-\infty$	$-\infty$	$-\infty$
6p24-p21.3	F13A	0.00	0.00	0.06	0.08	0.00
6p21.3-p21.1	GLO1	0.60	$-\infty$	$-\infty$	0.70	$-\infty$
6p21.3	BF	0.00	0.00	-2.07	-0.27	0.046
8q23	GPT	-2.3	$-\infty$	-0.32	$-\infty$	0.00
9q31-qter	ORM	0.29	0.00	0.35	-1.9	0.00
9q34.1-q34.2	ABO	$-\infty$	0.00	$-\infty$	$-\infty$	0.076
9q34.1-q34.2	AK1	0.00	0.00	0.008	-2.06	0.00
11p15.5	HBB*					
13q14.1-q14.2	ESD	$-\infty$	0.00	0.025	0.039	0.00
14q32.1	PI	0.00	0.30	-2.5	$-\infty$	0.29
15q11	p189-1*					
15q11	pIR4-3	$-\infty$	0.00	0.00	$-\infty$	0.00
15q11	pDX15	0.00	0.00	0.00	-0.29	*
15q14-q22	pDX50*					
16p13	PGP					
16q22	HP	$-\infty$	0.00	0.10	0.31	0.00
18q11-q12	Jk	-0.62	0.02	-0.43	0.70	-2.20
19q12-q13	Lu	0.00	$-\infty$	0.007	$-\infty$	0.007
19	Le	0.04	0.004	0.0185	0.117	-0.002
20	ADA	0.00	0.00	0.01	-0.42	0.00
22q11.2-qter	P1	0.18	0.029	0.013	0.12	-0.25
	KELL	0.00	0.00	0.011	$-\infty$	0.11

*Not polymorphic

(7.4%). Neither have we seen an increased frequency of autoimmune disease in these families (only one instance has been recorded in 26 affected and none in 13 unaffected relatives). The presence of atopic disorders (asthma, atopic dermatitis, hay fever) are also not different; 21/47 (45%) in dyslexic and 17/33 (52%) in non-dyslexic relatives. An initial battery of screening tests for autoimmune disease including antinuclear antibody (ANA) have not yielded positive results and have

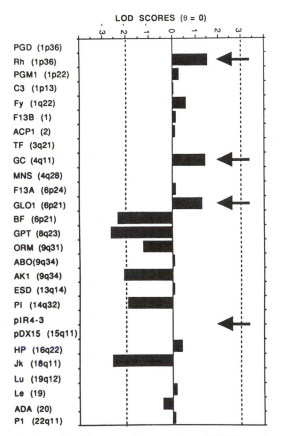

Figure 4. Graph of total LOD scores for protein and DNA markers. Data treatment is described in the text. Arrows indicate genomic loci targeted for further study.

been discontinued. An analysis of T-cell subsets, however, was also carried out and some of the results were unexpected. Cells that carry the monoclonal surface marker T4 are named *helper cells*, because they induce B-cells to make antibodies. Cells that carry the surface marker T8 are *suppressor cells*, which suppress, or turn off B-cell function. The majority of females with the gene for dyslexia in these families have an elevated T4/T8 lymphocyte ratio (figure 5). The clinical significance of this finding is unclear. These females may be more immunologically reactive although they were all clinically normal at the time of the study. The elevated T4/T8 ratios tended to cluster in two families and be unremarkable in others (figure 6). In Family 3015, two females warrant comment. The ratio was high in 3015-237, who was an unaffected obligate carrier. There remains the possibility that 3015-246, an apparently unaffected female with an elevated ratio, is actually a similarly unaf-

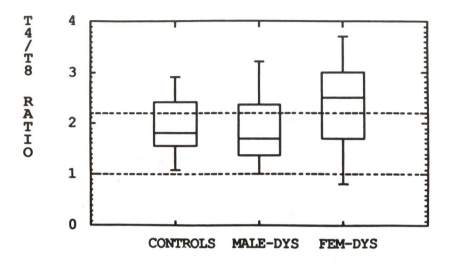

Figure 5.   Dotted lines indicate usual normal limits. Mean values are indicated by lines in boxes; boxes indicate one standard deviation. Female dyslexics have significantly higher values.

fected carrier and that the T4/T8 ratio was the only current indicator of her carrier status. More data are needed.

The general observation that the elevated T4/T8 ratio was found predominantly in affected females in certain families is of uncertain biological significance. Both the brain asymmetry in dyslexic females (to be discussed below) and these findings might result from early hormonal differences, as suggested by Geschwind and Galaburda (1985).

Vision and Auditory Studies.   Because reading involves both vision and language, we have undertaken studies of both processes using psychophysical methods that are sensitive enough to detect subtle abnormalities. Because dyslexics have clinically normal sensory function in both modalities, the problem is likely to be one that is more centrally located and involves a later stage of information processing in the brain. To study these "higher order" processes, it is of course necessary to rule out more peripheral sensory problems. We have accomplished this by providing visual and auditory screening exams that establish sensory function normality prior to participation in the psychophysical studies. We will discuss here the results of the visual studies only.

The vision-oculomotor screening examination in general yielded no differences between dyslexics and normal readers on most of the tests conducted. However, results of the visual psychophysical studies

FAMILY NO.   3015

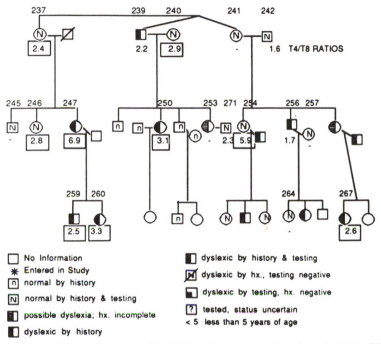

Figure 6.   T4/T8 ratios in Family 3015 with many high values (≥ 2.4). High values are shown in box under circle or squares.

differentiated visual performance of dyslexics and normal-reading adults. These studies are based on the concept of a two-channel visual system: a sustained, or pattern-detecting system, and the transient system, which is specialized for motion detection. These systems, roughly speaking, have their anatomical analogues in the parvocellular and magnocellular divisions of the visual system (Livingstone and Hubel 1987; Zeki and Shipp 1988). The sustained system is focal, and sensitive to patterns with high spatial resolution, i.e., small fine-grained objects such as letters. This system also has a slow temporal response, i.e., perception is not immediate. The transient system, which is designed to detect moving objects, often using peripheral vision, recognizes large objects having low spatial resolution. This system, although poor in spatial resolution, has fast temporal responses. The interaction between these two systems is probably critical in reading.

As one reads, the eye moves across the page in a series of saccades, interspersed with periods of visual fixation. During saccadic eye movements, vision is briefly suppressed, which prevents spatial overlapping of text information from one fixation to the next (Breitmeyer and Ganz 1976). This process may be thought of as a sort of beneficial masking of sustained system responses by activity in the transient system. However, if the period over which masking takes place is too long, reading might be impaired. This may be part of the problem encountered by some dyslexics.

To investigate a transient masking effect in the laboratory, we used a forward-masking paradigm. Figure 7 shows the time relationships between the mask and target. Targets to be detected were high or low spatial-frequency sine-wave gratings, presented on a video screen under computer control. Subjectively these patterns appeared as fuzzy horizontal stripes across the screen, the width of which defined the spatial frequency (high, narrow stripes; low, wide stripes). Contrast of the grating was varied according to a predetermined psychophysical procedure to assess the sensitivity of the observer under different conditions. We also varied how long the pattern remained on the screen (target duration) and whether or not it was preceded by a visual mask.

The results showed a very specific difference in visual sensitivity between dyslexic and normal-reader adults. Only when the to-be-detected target was a high spatial-frequency grating of brief exposure did the dyslexics show a significant reduction in contrast sensitivity, relative to normal readers. This was observed both with and without the mask. Using the two-channel model of visual information processing, we suspect that this finding indicates a slowness in responding of

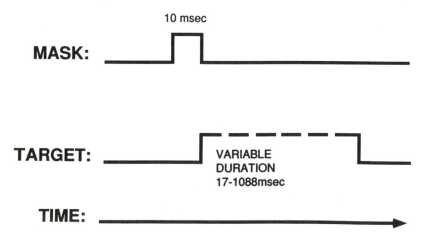

Figure 7. Time relationships between presentation of masking stimulus and a to-be-detected target, a sine-wave grating pattern of varying duration and spatial frequency.

the sustained visual channel. If it takes dyslexics longer to perceive detailed visual information (such as letters in a word), this might also make them more vulnerable to the sensory effects of masking by saccadic suppression. Studies are in progress to explore this hypothesis further.

In sum, our study adds support to the notion that some dyslexics have a temporal visual information processing deficit. As this is a rather specific disorder, it is not easily demonstrated except by sensitive laboratory procedures in which stimulus parameters are well-controlled. Similar differences have been observed when other psychophysical methods have been used to compare visual information processing in dyslexics and normal readers (see Gross and Rothenberg 1979 for a review of these studies).

The idea of a decrease in efficiency for perception of detailed visual information has a parallel in the auditory system, as some dyslexics have been shown to have difficulty in processing rapidly changing speech (Tallal 1980), as well as non-speech auditory information (McCrosky and Kidder 1980). Our multiple measurements of both visual and speech discrimination in the same individuals will indicate whether or not this temporal deficit is modality specific. Preliminary data on a small sample of dyslexic adults suggest that it may not be, at least for some individuals. More conclusive data will be provided by studies that are currently underway.

Neuropsychological Studies. These studies have been organized to test a wide range of cognitive abilities related to the reading and writing process (figure 8). Two approaches have been taken in the interpretation of these data. The first uses conventional statistics and compares the findings of dyslexic and non-dyslexic groups. The second approach involves inspection of the data by pedigree. These findings are summarized in table IV.

Since the number of children studied is still small, table IV includes only the adult comparisons. This approach allows for the detection of statistically significant differences, and allows the geneticist to determine whether positive results are due to random variation or whether certain families are unremarkable while most of the positive tests occurred in other families. Both approaches are valid, but have different strengths and limitations.

The results of several tests can be presented in this fashion. The FAS test measures verbal fluency by requiring the subjects to name as many words as possible beginning with the letter F, A, and S. The number of words are individually recorded and summed. Overall, 33 words were given by unaffected adults compared to 45 for dyslexics ($p = .01$). This was an unexpected result, not observed in prior developmental studies. Similarly, the Menyuk Syntactic Comprehension

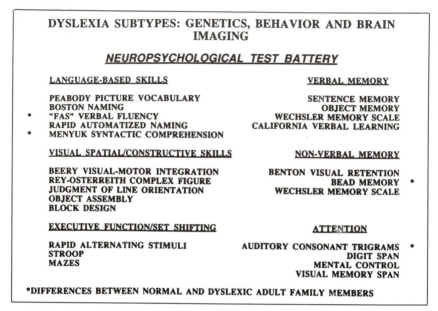

DYSLEXIA SUBTYPES: GENETICS, BEHAVIOR AND BRAIN IMAGING

NEUROPSYCHOLOGICAL TEST BATTERY

LANGUAGE-BASED SKILLS

PEABODY PICTURE VOCABULARY
BOSTON NAMING
• "FAS" VERBAL FLUENCY
RAPID AUTOMATIZED NAMING
• MENYUK SYNTACTIC COMPREHENSION

VISUAL SPATIAL/CONSTRUCTIVE SKILLS

BEERY VISUAL-MOTOR INTEGRATION
REY-OSTERREITH COMPLEX FIGURE
JUDGMENT OF LINE ORIENTATION
OBJECT ASSEMBLY
BLOCK DESIGN

EXECUTIVE FUNCTION/SET SHIFTING

RAPID ALTERNATING STIMULI
STROOP
MAZES

VERBAL MEMORY

SENTENCE MEMORY
OBJECT MEMORY
WECHSLER MEMORY SCALE
CALIFORNIA VERBAL LEARNING

NON-VERBAL MEMORY

BENTON VISUAL RETENTION
BEAD MEMORY •
WECHSLER MEMORY SCALE

ATTENTION

AUDITORY CONSONANT TRIGRAMS •
DIGIT SPAN
MENTAL CONTROL
VISUAL MEMORY SPAN

•DIFFERENCES BETWEEN NORMAL AND DYSLEXIC ADULT FAMILY MEMBERS

Figure 8. The various neuropsychological tests are noted according to the cognitive domain tested.

Test, also given verbally, yielded unexpected results. A simple statement is given, such as: "The lion that the tiger bit, jumped over the giraffe." The subject is asked "Who jumped over the giraffe?" Answer: "The lion." On this task, dyslexics did less well than normals ($p = .001$), a finding suggesting difficulty handling embedded syntactic markers. The Auditory Consonant Trigrams test also yielded unexpected and possibly very significant results. Three-letter meaningless trigrams (words with no vowels) are presented (example: LDX) and the subjects are asked to either recite the trigram immediately or to count backwards for 3, 9, then 18 seconds before repeating the three letters. This task becomes difficult at 9 seconds and, by 18 seconds, it is quite hard. At 9 seconds and at 18 seconds, and for the total scores, the scores were significantly different between the 18 normals and 16 dyslexics ($p < .03$). This suggests that dyslexics may have difficulty ignoring competing stimuli that interfere with immediate recall.

The second approach, which involved inspection of the data by pedigree, also gave quite interesting results. This review was greatly facilitated by developing a system for storing more than 400 variables on each family member in a MacIntosh computer system programmed to select up to 4 variables to be printed out below each appropriate circle or square (figures 9 and 10). The person's pedigree number is above the circle or square (413, 411, 418, etc. in figure 10). The totals for the

Table IV. Summary of Significant T-Test Results on Adult (>18 Yrs.) Family Members

			Language Based Skills		ΣN	
					D	N
(Verbal Fluency				Normal		
FAS Test)			Dyslexics (D)	Readers (N)		
	F	p = .027	16 ± 6 >	12 ± 4	16	18
	A	p = .019	13 ± 6 >	9 ± 3	16	18
	S	p = .001	17 ± 5 >	11 ± 4	16	18
	Total	p = .010	45 ± 16 >	33 ± 11	16	18

Visual-Spatial/Constructive Skills

				Normal		
(Beery Visual			Dyslexics	Readers		
Motor-Integration)		p = .036	21 ± 2 <	22 ± 2	16	18
(Rey Osterreith						
Complex Diagram)		p = .046	34.6 ± 1.5 <	35.5 ± 9	15	17

Verbal Memory Skills

				Normal		
			Dyslexics	Readers		
(Menyuk Syntactic						
Comprehension)		p = .001	12 ± 2 <	15 ± 2	16	18
				Normal		
			Dyslexics	Readers		
(Auditory	9 secs.	p = .038	2 ± 1 <	3 ± 2	16	18
Consonant	18 secs.	p = .003	.8 ± 1 <	2 ± 1	16	18
Trigrams)	Total	p = .029	12 ± 3 <	15 ± 4	16	18

dyslexics in this pedigree are shown with a box around them (63, 68, etc.). The two normals scored 38 and 27 words respectively, which was comparable to other normals. The average for the dyslexics, however, was 58. The data from this family account for all of the difference shown in table IV. Clearly, in this family the dyslexics have remarkably good verbal fluency. This is especially interesting since many people with dyslexia do extremely well in real life, particularly in business. Increased verbal fluency may be part of the explanation for this observation, at least in a subgroup of families, and more data are needed to validate this observation.

When pedigree data were inspected, similar results occurred in two other tests: the Menyuk Test and Auditory Consonant Trigrams. Two families (3001 and 3015) did poorly with Auditory Consonant Trigrams. Menyuk Test results are shown for one family in figure 9. Other families were unremarkable. Together these results provide important preliminary evidence of behavioral differences between families and indirectly for genetic heterogeneity, with several different genes producing important and previously unrecognized differences in the phenotype(s) associated with dyslexia in adults.

FAMILY NO.   3015

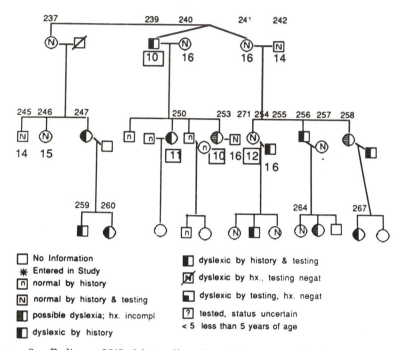

□ No Information	▉ dyslexic by history & testing
✳ Entered in Study	▨ dyslexic by hx., testing negat
⊡ normal by history	▉ dyslexic by testing, hx. negat
Ⓝ normal by history & testing	[?] tested, status uncertain
▤ possible dyslexia; hx. incompl	< 5 less than 5 years of age
◧ dyslexic by history	

Figure 9.   Pedigree 3015. Most affected members scored below the overall mean dyslexic performance on the Menyuk Syntactic Comprehensive Test, as well as below unaffected family members. The low scores for the Menyuk Syntactic Comprehension Test are shown in the boxes under the circles and squares.

Magnetic Resonance Imaging (MRI) Studies.   We have used positron-emission tomography (PET) (Gross-Glenn et al. 1986) and magnetic resonance imaging (MRI) to study localization of the putative neural substrate for dyslexia. Following Galaburda's post-mortem studies of dyslexic brains (Galaburda et al. 1985), others (using MRI) have noted symmetry of the planum temporale in dyslexics, rather than the usual L > R asymmetry for this region (Hynd et al. in press; Larsen et al. in press). As we have found this region difficult to measure reliably, we have taken an approach that involves measuring clearly specified brain areas on a cross-sectional plane that transects many of the regions thought to be important for reading. Since behavioral studies have suggested possible deficits for dyslexics in interhemispheric transmission of neural signals, we have also measured the cross-sectional area of the corpus callosum (Gross-Glenn et al. 1989).

FAMILY NO. 3017

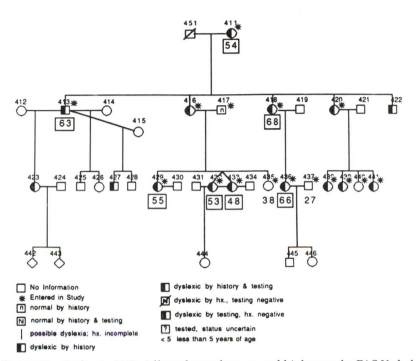

Figure 10.   Pedigree 3017. Affected members scored higher on the FAS Verbal Fluency Test compared to overall unaffected members across all families. The high scores for the FAS Verbal Fluency Test are shown in the boxes under the circles and squares.

Twenty-one dyslexic and thirty non-dyslexic right-handed adults were studied by MRIs. Approximately 15% were members of families in the present studies, and the remaining were ascertained according to similar criteria. IQ was verified, and there existed both a childhood and a family history of reading and spelling difficulties in at least two generations. A diagnosis of developmental dyslexia in adults was made if there was a 1.5 standard deviation discrepancy between full scale IQ and performance on reading and spelling tests.

MRI studies were carried out with a Siemens Magnetom scanner (1.0 or 1.5 Tesla) at a slice thickness of 7.0 mm with 3.0 mm interslice intervals. Sagittal T1-weighted spin echo sequences (TR 500ms, TE 17ms) and transverse T2-weighted spin echo sequences (TR 2500ms, TE 25ms and 90ms) were used.

Planimetric area measurements (in cm²) were derived from hand tracings of MRI scans. Horizontal areas were measured from transverse MRI scans at the level of the Foramen of Monro, containing the plane transecting the basal ganglia and the four tips of the lateral ventricle horns. As shown in figure 11, a midline axis was drawn from the anterior to the posterior aspect of the interhemispheric fissure. Based on the linear extension of this midline axis, the cross-sectional area of this plane was divided into six regions: anterior and posterior 10%, plus four 20% regions between these poles. A laterality index (LI) was calculated using the absolute cross-sectional areas for each region: $LI = (R - L) \times 200/(R + L)$ (R = right area, L = left area).

Corpus callosum cross-section area was measured from scans taken in the midsagittal plane. The corpus callosum was traced directly and divided linearly from anterior to posterior (figure 12). Areas of the anterior fifth (genu), posterior fifth (splenium), and middle ⅗ section were normalized to the midsagittal brain area to control for differences in brain size. Two-way ANOVAs were performed on mean values of the areas measured, with sex and diagnosis being the constant factors.

Results of the MRI studies can be summarized briefly here. As shown in figure 11, there was a general progression from $R > L$ asymmetry anteriorly to $L > R$ asymmetry posteriorly in both groups. This pattern is consistent with previously reported cerebral asymmetries (Weinberger et al. 1982; Chui and Damasio 1980; LeMay and Kido 1978). The only region in which cerebral asymmetry for dyslexics and normals differed was the mid-posterior region, an area that encompasses the angular gyrus of the inferior parietal lobe. Here, dyslexics showed a $R > L$ hemispheric asymmetry in contrast to the $L > R$ pat-

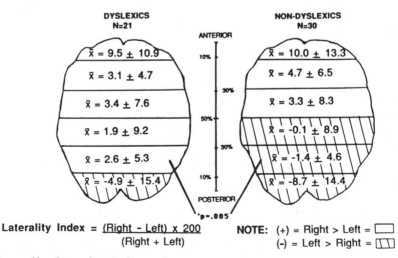

Figure 11. Laterality indices of transverse brain areas obtained from MRI scans at the level of the Foramen of Monro. Right > left asymmetry of the mid-posterior region for dyslexics was significantly different from the left right pattern of asymmetry observed here for normal readers.

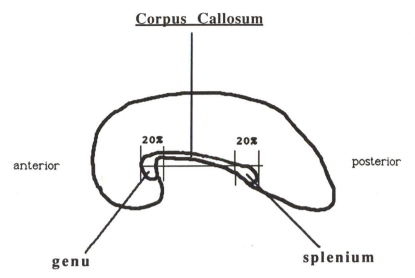

Corpus Callosum

anterior   posterior

genu   **splenium**

Figure 12.   Sagittal area tracing of the corpus callosum, and midsagittal brain area to illustrate measurements taken from MRI scans. Areas of callosal regions were normalized to individual's midsagittal brain area.

tern observed in normal readers in the midposterior region (F = 8.7, p = .005). Group differences were also noted in the callosal area with dyslexics showing a relatively larger splenium than normal readers (F = 8.9, p = .005) (see table V). Much of this difference was due to female dyslexics, who also showed a significantly larger genu and total corpus callosum area than the other groups.

Positron-Emission Tomographic Studies.   PET-scan studies were carried out on 25 right-handed adult male volunteers. The subject was

Table V.   Normalized Mean Corpus Callosum Cross-Section Area Measurements 20 Dyslexics (D) Versus 30 Non-Dyslexics (N)

	genu				splenium				total		
	♀	♂	X̄		♀	♂	X̄		♀	♂	X̄
D	.024	.019	.021	D	.022	.018	.020	D	.075	.064	.069
N	.020	.020	.020	N	.018	.017	.017	N	.065	.066	.066
X̄	.021	.020		X̄	.020	.017		X̄	.069	.065	

Interaction
Diagnosis x Sex
(F = 6.4, p = .015)

Diagnosis (F = 8.9, p = .005)
Sex (F = 7.9, p = .007)
Interaction
Diagnosis x Sex
(F = 3.1, p = .085)

Interaction
Diagnosis x Sex
(F = 5.8, p = .020)

given an injection of a glucose analog, 2-deoxyglucose, which is labeled with a very short-lived isotope of fluorine (F-18). The brain initially utilizes this substance (FDG) as though it were glucose and it becomes concentrated in areas of the brain that are metabolically active over a 30-minute period. During this time, the subject read aloud a list of simple words. Following this activation period, the subject was scanned to reveal brain regions of varying metabolic activity, based on the PET camera's detection of the regional uptake of FDG.

PET studies have been carried out in a relatively small number of study families as well as a sample of other familial dyslexics and normal readers. Dyslexia was diagnosed according to the same criteria as for the MRI studies (see above). Similar to other studies during reading (Petersen et al. 1988), we found that a simple reading task produced wide-spread variations in metabolic activity in many brain regions. Significant differences in normalized metabolic activity between dyslexics and normal readers were localized to prefontal and inferior visual (lingual) regions (Duara et al. 1989; Gross-Glenn et al. in press).

Compared with normal readers, dyslexics showed a reversal of the L > R pattern of metabolic asymmetry in the lingual region. This region is part of the occipito-temporal pathway that has been shown in monkeys to be important for identification of complex visual patterns (Mishkin, Ungerleider, and Macko 1983; Ungerleider and Mishkin 1982). In the prefrontal region, dyslexics showed more symmetry than the R > L asymmetry observed in normal readers. Evidence from both animal and human studies suggests that prefrontal cortex plays an important role in temporal and cross-modal integration of behavior (Fuster 1985; Pandya and Yeterian 1985).

In order to determine whether metabolic and anatomic asymmetries in these regions correspond in the same individuals, we measured prefrontal and lingual areas from multi-slice horizontal MRI scans on 16 subjects having both types of scans. For normal readers, direction of asymmetry matched; for dyslexics, however, a significant number of subjects showed a "mismatch" between PET and MRI in the lingual region ($\chi^2 = 5.69$, $p < .02$) (figure 13). Prefrontal cortex showed a similar, but nonsignificant ($p = .08$) trend (figure 14). Usually the mismatch resulted from aberrant PET (rather than MRI) findings. This suggests that metabolic differences related to reading in dyslexics are not simply related to differences in gross structural anatomy. Despite this result, reversed anatomic asymmetry (R > L) for these dyslexics was observed more dorsally in the inferior parietal lobe as was found in the MRI studies on a larger group of subjects (see above).

Twenty-six of the subjects who underwent the visual psychophysical studies also participated in the MRI studies. To study the relationship between cerebral asymmetry and visual performance we correlated laterality indices derived from MRI measurements with performance on

LINGUAL REGION LATERALITY INDICES

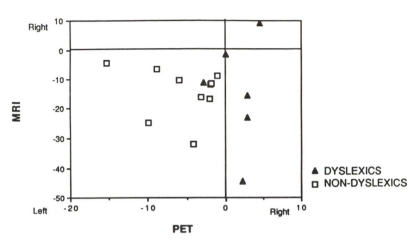

Figure 13. Plot of PET and MRI laterality indices for lingual regions showing clustering of normals to left on both measurements. In dyslexics left > right MRI asymmetry was not usually matched by direction of metabolic asymmetry on PET-scans.

the visual psychophysical study described above. The most significant finding in this vision study was dyslexics' elevated thresholds for detection of short duration high spatial frequency information, especially when targets were preceded by a mask.

To characterize each subject's masking vulnerability in this condition, we calculated a duration at which visual sensitivity was decreased by a factor of two. Long durations indicate less sensitivity as the target required more time for perception. In figure 15 this aspect of performance has been plotted on the x-axis. On the y-axis is plotted each subject's MRI laterality index for mid-posterior regions in which the two groups were found to differ. With one exception among dyslexics, those with the poorest visual performance also showed R > L asymmetry in this region (see upper right quadrant). The two measures were positively correlated in the combined group ($r = .41$, $p = .02$). Taken together, PET, MRI, and visual psychophysical studies suggest a difference in visual-system functioning for dyslexics, perhaps localized to extra-striate regions adjacent to temporal and inferior parietal cortex.

DISCUSSION

One likely outcome of these studies should be the development of both genetic and functional tests for each of the (presumed) types of dyslexia. There is now no single functional test for dyslexia and this has

PREFRONTAL REGION LATERALITY INDICES

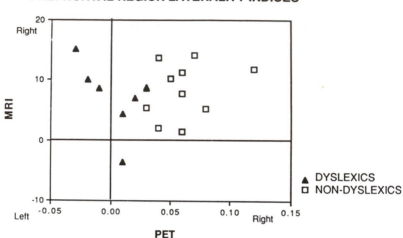

Figure 14.   Plot of PET and MRI laterality indices for prefrontal region, show-ing a clustering of normals and some dyslexics with right > left asymmetry on both measures. Several dyslexics however failed to show this correspondence between measurements.

been a significant impediment to research. The lack of such a test has undoubtedly led to the selection of widely different study samples (all called "dyslexia"), but whose results then cannot really be compared. Several stages of genetic studies can be predicted. With a series of link-

MRI ASYMMETRY vs. VISUAL PERFORMANCE

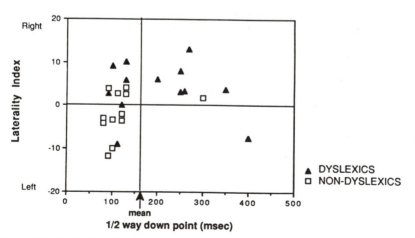

Figure 15.   Individual subjects' laterality indices obtained from MRI measure-ments of midposterior region (figure 11) are plotted against each subjects' sus-ceptibility to visual masking of high spatial-frequency patterns. Longer dura-tions on the x-axis indicate a stronger masking effect and reduced sensitivity.

age studies resulting in more closely linked markers, we ultimately should be able to localize and isolate the gene(s), just as has been done for Duchenne muscular dystrophy and cystic fibrosis. Then we will have a simple, direct test for each type that will not require family studies, and that can be done at birth, or even before birth. This will provide an opportunity for both observing and introducing alternative forms of remediation early in life or different approaches to school. In a few years, it should be possible either to avoid many of the emotional and school problems that these children have or to alleviate them. The family history, in the interval, is critical, and asking about a history of dyslexia should be part of the school admission process. Recognition of the fact that a child should be specifically evaluated for dyslexia when there is a family history of dyslexia, should lead to early testing and make a major difference to many children. Eventually it is likely that different remediation strategies will be appropriate for different types of familial dyslexia.

SUMMARY AND CONCLUSION

There is a significant subgroup of children and adults with autosomal dominant inheritance of dyslexia, and the pedigrees and other data in this study provide additional evidence in support of this observation. Penetrance is greater than 90%, a value consistent with other autosomal dominantly inherited disorders. The frequency remains unknown, because we do not yet have a specific test, but is probably high. Clearly, it is not rare. There is also, now, significant evidence for genetic heterogeneity both from the genetic studies and the observation of phenotypic differences between families in the present study. These variant genes must have been present 10,000 years ago, long before reading and writing began. There may well have been advantages or disadvantage to these genes, having nothing to do with reading both then and now, and the present study has shown at least one possible advantage in verbal fluency.

The male-female differences remain challenging. The present evidence suggests that the reported excess of males is not biologically correct since the sex ratio is not different from 1.0 in these families; rather, females are less severely affected and less often recognized. There is likely an interaction between the gene(s) for dyslexia, sex hormones, and possibly even concomitantly caused immunologic responses in the development of brains in dyslexia, that requires much more data and study before a clear picture emerges. The linkage studies, however, have not as yet yielded a clearly confirmed linkage, but there is good evidence that several genes are involved; the most promising linkage studies suggest that there are genes leading to dyslexia on chromosomes 15 and 6. The PET, MRI, vision, speech perception, and neuro-psychological studies are all extremely promising and have given highly suggestive evidence of "clinical" heterogeneity. They may result in the identification of parameters by which the (presumed) several genes may be measured functionally. Methods are available for resolution of the overall problem, but because of its complexity many more families need to be studied. A very different view of the mechanisms resulting in the phenotype(s) of dyslexia and what we might do about them should evolve from this and related studies over the next five to ten years.

REFERENCES

Bisgaard, M. L., Eiberg, H., Moller, N., Niebuhr, E., and Mohr, J. 1987. Dyslexia and chromosome 15 heteromorphism: Negative lod score in a Danish material. *Clinical Genetics* 32:118–119.

Breitmeyer, B. G., and Ganz, L. 1976. Implications of sustained and transient channels for theories of visual pattern masking, saccadic suppression, and information processing. *Psychological Review* 83:1–36.

Chui, H. C., and Damasio, A. R. 1980. Human cerebral asymmetries evaluated by computed tomography. *Journal of Neurology, Neurosurgery and Psychiatry* 43:873–78.

Duara, R., Gross-Glenn, K., Barker, W., Loewenstein, D., Chang, J. Y., Apicella, A., Yoshii, F., Pascal, S., and Lubs, H. A. 1989. PET studies during reading in dyslexics and controls. *Neurology* 39(suppl. 1):165.

Finucci, J. M., Guthrie, J. T., Childs, A. L., Abbey, H., and Childs, B. 1976. The genetics of specific reading disability. *Annals of Human Genetics* 40:1–23.

Fuster, J. M. 1985. The prefrontal cortex and temporal integration. In *Cerebral Cortex, Association and Auditory Cortices,* eds. A. Peters and E. G. Jones. New York: Plenum Press.

Galaburda, A. M., Sherman, G. F., Rosen, G. D., Aboitiz, F., and Geschwind, N. 1985. Developmental dyslexia: Four consecutive patients with cortical anomalies. *Annals of Neurology* 18:222–33.

Geschwind, N., and Galaburda, A. M. 1985. Cerebral lateralization—Biological mechanisms, associations, and pathology: II. A hypothesis and a program for research. *Archives of Neurology* 45:521–52.

Gross, K., and Rothenberg, S. 1979. An examination of methods used to test the visual perceptual deficit hypothesis of dyslexia. *Journal of Learning Disabilities* 12(9):670–77.

Gross-Glenn, K., Coleman-Lewis, D., Smith, S. D., and Lubs, H. A. 1985. Phenotype of adult familial dyslexia: Reading of visually transformed texts and nonsense passages. *International Journal of Neuroscience* 28:49–59.

Gross-Glenn, K., Duara, R., Barker, W., Loewenstein, D., Chang, J.-Y., Yoshii, F., Apicella, A., Pascal, S., Boothe, T., Sevush, S., Jallad, B., Novoa, L., and Lubs, H. in press. Positron emission tomographic studies during serial word-reading by normal and dyslexic adults. *Journal of Clinical Experimental Neuropsychology.*

Gross-Glenn, K., Duara, R., Yoshii, F., Barker, W., Chen, Y., Apicella, A., Boothe, T., and Lubs, H. 1986. PET-scan studies during reading in dyslexia and non-dyslexic adults. *Society for Neuroscience, Abstracts* 12(part 2):1364.

Gross-Glenn, K., Duara, R., Kushch, A., Pascal, S., Barker, W., Jallad, B., and Lubs, H. A. 1989. MRI and visual psychophysical studies of inherited dyslexia. *Society for Neuroscience Abstracts* 15(1):482.

Gross-Glenn, K., Jallad, B., Novoa, L., Helgren-Lempesis, V., and Lubs, H. A. 1990. Nonsense Passage reading as an aid to the diagnosis of familial dyslexia in adults. *Reading and Writing: An Interdisciplinary Journal* 2:149–61.

Hynd, G. W., Semrud-Clikeman, M., Lorys, A. R., Novey, E. S., and Eliopulos, D. (in press). Brain morphology in developmental dyslexia and attention deficit disorder/hyperactivity. *Archives of Neurology.*

Larsen, J. P., Hoien, T., Lundberg, I., and Odegaard, H. in press. MRI Evaluation of the size and symmetry of the planum temporale in adolescents with developmental dyslexia. *Brain and Language.*

LeMay, M., and Kido, D. K. 1978. Asymmetries of the cerebral hemispheres on computed tomograms. *Journal of Computer Assisted Tomography* 2:471–76.

Livingstone, M., and Hubel, D. 1987. Psychophysical evidence for separate channels for the perception of form, color, movement, and depth. *Journal of Neuroscience* 7(11):3416–68.

Lubs, H. A., Rabin, M., Carland-Saucier, K., Wen, X. L., Gross-Glenn, K., Duara, R., Levin, B., and Lubs, M. L. 1990. Genetic bases of developmental dyslexia: Molecular studies. In *Neuropsychological Foundations of Learning Disabilities: A Handbook of Issues, Methods and Practice*, eds. J. Obrzut and G. Hynd. Orlando, FL: Academic Press, Inc.

McCroskey, R., and Kidder, H. 1980. Auditory fusion among learning disabled, reading disabled and normal children. *Journal of Learning Disabilities* 13(2):18–25.

Mishkin, M., Ungerleider, L. G., and Macko, K. A. 1983. Object vision and spatial vision: Two cortical pathways. *Trends in Neuroscience* 6:414–17.

Pandya, D. N., and Yeterian, E. 1985. Architecture and connections of cortical association areas. In *Cerebral Cortex Association and Auditory Cortices*, eds. A. Peters and E. G. Jones 4:3–61. New York: Plenum Press.

Petersen, S. E., Fox, P. T., Posner, M. I., Minton, M., and Raichle, M. E. 1988. Positron emission tomographic studies of the cortical anatomy of single-word processing. *Nature* 331:585–589.

Smith, S. D., Kimberling, W. J., Pennington, B. F., and Lubs, H. A. 1983. Specific reading disability: Identification of an inherited form through linkage analysis. *Science* 219:1345–47.

Smith, S. D., Pennington, B. F., Kimberling, W. J., and Ing, P. S. 1990a. Familial dyslexia: Use of genetic linkage data to define subtypes. *American Academy of Child and Adolescent Psychiatry* 29(2):204–13.

Smith, S. D., Pennington, B. F., Kimberling, W. J., and Ing, P. S. 1990b. Genetic linkage analysis with specific dyslexia: Use of multiple markers to include and exclude possible loci. In *Perspectives on Dyslexia*, Vol. 1, ed. G. Th. Pavlidis. New York: John Wiley & Sons Ltd.

Tallal, P. 1980. Auditory temporal perception phonics and reading disabilities in children. *Brain and Language* 9(2):182–98.

Ungerlieder, L. G., Mishkin, M. 1982. Two cortical visual systems. In *Analysis of Visual Behavior*, eds. D. J. Ingle, M. A. Goodale, and R. J. W. Mansfield. Cambridge, MA: The MIT Press.

Weinberger, D. R., Luchins, D. J., Morihisa, J., and Wyatt, R. J. 1982. Asymmetrical volumes of the right and left frontal and occipital regions of the human brain. *Annals of Neurology* 11:97–100.

Zeki, S., and Shipp, S. 1988. The functional logic of cortical connections. *Nature* 335:311–17.

Chapter • 5

Anatomy of Dyslexia
Argument
Against Phrenology

Albert M. Galaburda

Behavioral neurology and neuropsychology (BN/NP) are collaborating clinical fields that deal with neurologic explanations of behavior, both normal and abnormal. One of the basic assumptions of these fields is that for each behavior, cognitive or emotional, there is a discoverable underlying brain mechanism, and the corollary assumption is that defective behavior denotes a defect in the underlying brain machinery that subserves that behavior.

The theories and methodologies associated with BN/NP have developed over nearly 200 years, and reflect still to a large extent, phrenologic influences of the mid-nineteenth century. At the start of the nineteenth century, the way to view the brain was bound to change. This is because the introduction of chromate salts to fix (harden) the brain after death made reproducible dissection possible for the first time. Most of the gross anatomic structures with which we are familiar now—gyri, sulci, lobes, and white matter bundles—were named and described during that time. The inevitable conclusion from the rapidly growing knowledge of brain anatomy was that the brain was not "a bowl of jello," but rather an organized structure containing consistent, discrete areas interconnected in consistent, discrete patterns via fiber pathways. From this—as well as from early experiments on stimula-

Some of the research reported here was supported by NIH grants HD 20806, HD 19819, by a grant from the Carl W. Herzog Foundation, and by a grant from the Research Division of The Orton Dyslexia Society.

tion of parts of the cortex and observations on the delimited effects of brain injury—it was not difficult for workers of that time to conclude that discrete anatomical regions subserved discrete functions. Phrenology was nothing more than the extrapolation of specific markings on the brain to protuberances on the surface of the cranium, the assumption being that well developed cerebral surface structures indent the cranium from the inside and produce such protuberances; hence cranial markings could also predict specific functions.

The best known contributor to our early knowledge about the effects of focal brain damage on delimited functional loss, in this case language (speech) function, is Paul Broca, a follower of the phrenologic school. He described the first widely recognized patient with a left frontal lobe lesion resulting in aphasia. Interestingly, in turn, was the fact that Broca was very active in the emerging field of physical anthropology, which bases its scientific claims on metric measurements of anatomic structures. The concept that greater intellectual capacity reflects greater cranial capacity arose from physical anthropology, which compared the endocranial volumes of apes, and fossil and extant humans; thus, it was assumed that humans had the greatest intellectual development in the animal kingdom because their cranial contents were the largest by comparison to the body size, suggesting therefore that *bigger is better*. Physical anthropology, at least through Broca, had a human link to the phrenologists of the nineteenth century, who also claimed that bigger is better. For instance, people with prominent eyes were thought to be eloquent, which reflected the fact that prominent eyes may result from shallow-built orbits, which in turn meant that the frontal lobes were greatly developed and pushed the orbits from behind!

The study of brain asymmetries was motivated in part by the concept of bigger is better. It was argued that since the left hemisphere was implicated in language functions, then it should be larger, at least in the portions that participate in those functions. Initially workers weighed and otherwise metrically compared the hemispheres as wholes. No doubt disappointingly to the workers of that time, no consistent differences between the hemispheres were found. Near the end of the nineteenth century, the Sylvian fissures, around which brain regions involved in language function are found, were described to be asymmetric (see Galaburda et al. 1978). But, to my knowledge, it was not until the 1930s that the asymmetry of greatest concern to us, that of the planum temporale, was first noted (see Geschwind and Levitsky 1968). Discussion about the brain as an interesting source of behavior, together with descriptions of the functional anatomy of the brain, including brain asymmetries, began to wane soon after WWI, to be replaced by the emerging power of psychological explanations. The interest lived on within the small and arcane field of neuropsychiatry, which in the '60s and '70s gave way to behavioral neurology and neuropsychology.

One of the reasons for the premature demise of the phrenologic approach to the neurology of behavior, which may be of particular interest to the readers of this chapter, came from the confusion presented by lesions occurring in childhood (see Lenneberg 1967). Children often failed to demonstrate standard behavioral syndromes from the exact brain lesions that caused them in adult life. In fact children sometimes showed no deficits whatsoever! This led to the conclusion that there was much more "equipotentiality" of brain organization, not nearly as discrete as would be inferred from phrenologic teaching, such that one area of the brain could substitute for another—at least in the case of damage. This kind of functional "plasticity" did throw into question the tenets of classical neuropyschology, and, unfortunately, not enough was as yet known about cognitive science or developmental brain plasticity to permit the conclusion that both localization and the ability to adjust to damage, at least in part, could be acceptable to a coherent understanding of brain/behavior relationships. So, neuropsychology suffered temporarily.

Norman Geschwind was perhaps the single most important figure in contemporary neurology to influence the revival of neuropsychological explanations of behavior in the United States. This revival began in the early 1960s and was characterized by a resurgence in the emphasis on localization of lesions and the deficits they produced, description of discrete connecting pathways, and the study of brain asymmetry. Geschwind and Levitsky (1968) reported on the distribution of asymmetry of the planum temporale in neurologically intact brains. In this landmark study, brains were found to exhibit asymmetry in favor of the planum temporale of the left hemisphere, an area implicated in language function because it contains regions of cortex where lesions may cause language disorders. The larger left planum temporale, found in over ⅔ of brains, was taken to explain the superiority of the left hemisphere in language tasks and the vulnerability of that side to the production of aphasia by lesions in the area of the planum. Moreover, Geschwind suggested that the left planum might be small on both sides in children with developmental language disorders, for instance, dyslexia (Geschwind 1968). Indeed, a similar suggestion had been provided by the late-nineteenth–turn-of-the-century theories on "congenital word blindness" of Hinshelwood (1917). These theories implicate incomplete development of the posterior left parietal regions in acquired reading disorders following the work of the French neurologist and follower of Broca—Jules Déjérine (1892).

In 1978, when I was encouraged by Norman Geschwind to analyze the brain of a dyslexic man, the hypothesis to be tested was that both the left and right plana temporale would be developmentally small, thus confirming the phrenologic hypothesis. This did not turn out to be the case. The brain showed instead the form of symmetry of the planum temporale ordinarily seen in 25% of normative brains (see below). In addition, the same brain showed focal abnormalities of the cortical architecture of, predominantly, the left perisylvian regions. As I will point out in the following pages, both findings—symmetry and the cortical anomalies—would argue against the traditional phrenologic interpretation of brain-behavior relationships.

THE MEANING OF SYMMETRY

After the original case report, our laboratory analyzed a total of six male and three female brains from dyslexic individuals and found all of them to show symmetry of the planum temporale (Galaburda 1988). This represents a statistically unexpected finding, since symmetric plana occur in only about a fourth of the population—a third, were the population to be made up entirely of lefthanders (see Hochberg and LeMay 1975). Furthermore, there were earlier reports of aberrancy in the sample distribution of posterior cerebral asymmetry among dyslexic subjects studied by computerized tomographic (CT) scans. In normative series most scans show prominence of the left occipital region over the right. In the dyslexic subjects there was increased incidence of reversed asymmetry (right over left; Hier et al. 1978) or increased incidence of symmetry (Haslam et al. 1981). A number of ongoing studies (for instance, Jernigan, Hesselink, and Tallal 1989), some of which are reported in this symposium (Lubs et al., this volume; Lubs et al. 1988), and the work of Lundberg and Toien in Scandinavia (personal communication), have found symmetry in brain regions that include the planum temporale in populations of dyslexic subjects studied by magnetic resonance imaging. It appears, therefore, that more symmetry or otherwise an alteration in the standard pattern of asymmetry of the planum and related parts of the brain is statistically linked to, and can possibly be a causative factor in the learning disorder.

Does the presence of symmetry of a language area in the dyslexic subjects mean that dyslexics have two symmetric but small language areas, and therefore are "phrenologically" vulnerable to linguistic weakness? As already stated, the form of symmetry seen in the planum temporale of dyslexic brains is comparable to that seen in any brain with symmetric plana, and therefore consists of two large plana. Thus in ordinary brains, we found that the size of the planum temporale behaves in a specific way with respect to the *degree* of asymmetry of this structure (Galaburda et al. 1987); the greater the asymmetry, the smaller the total area occupied by the left and right planum together. In other words, symmetric plana, when measured together, are larger overall than asymmetric plana, and the symmetric plana of the dyslexic brains correspond in size to the large symmetric plana of ordinary brains. Furthermore, we found that the asymmetric case is not smaller than the symmetric case as a result of both sides being smaller. Instead, the left planum is comparable in size in asymmetric and symmetric cases, and only the right planum is smaller (except for a small percentage of ordinary brains in which the right planum is large and the left is small). Therefore, brains of dyslexic subjects do not have a small left hemisphere language area; instead, they have a large right hemisphere language area. We must therefore consider that, if symmetry plays any causative role in the linguistic deficit of developmental dyslexia, bigger is not necessarily better, and, therefore, this finding constitutes a blow to the phrenologic explanation of developmental dyslexia.

The planum temporale is a heterogeneous structure that contains several architectonic areas having different anatomic relationships and functions (Galaburda and Sanides 1980), which makes it unsuitable for asking detailed questions about histologic aspects of brain asymmetry. Therefore, the finding of asymmetry in other species offers a way for answering the question "What cellular features make a symmetric cortical area larger than an asymmetric one?" For instance, there may be more neurons in the symmetric case; or, conversely, there may be a comparable number of neurons that are larger (and farther apart); or a combination of different numbers and sizes of neurons, glia, connective tissues, blood vessels, and myelination. It is important to determine which factor plays the crucial role, since the answer would help pinpoint the developmental step during which anatomic asymmetry is determined and thus the time in which the dyslexic brain begins to differentiate from the ordinary brain.

Answering this question is not a simple matter in human brains because of limited availability of normative specimens and the enormously long process of parceling the large human architectonic areas. Fortunately however, symmetry and asymmetry of cerebral regions also are expressed in brains of nonhuman animals, which makes this task possible. However, a confusion that is common in this field must be dispelled first, since many have questioned the usefulness of animal models for characteristics that are thought to be typically "human."

There are at least two issues about asymmetry we need to consider: one relates to the question "To what extent is one side larger (or better?) than the other?"; the other relates to the question "Are more individuals in a given sample lateralized to the left or to the right?" Available research appears to show that these two issues are biologically distinct, and ought not to be lumped together in studies of hemispheric specialization and anatomic asymmetry. For instance, humans are highly lateralized for handedness, in that usually for each person one hand is consistently preferred over the other for most tasks; also, the distribution of handedness in all known normal human populations is biased, in that most people consistently prefer the right hand over the left. Individual rats and other animals, on the other hand, often show preference for one paw, but in a sample, roughly fifty percent prefer the right and fifty percent prefer the left paw. Furthermore, although it is possible to breed rats for strength of paw preference, directionality, i.e., left or right pawedness, does not breed (Collins 1981). Also, the presence of autoimmunity in mice alters the strength, but not the directionality, of asymmetry of certain cortical areas (Rosen et al. 1989a). Therefore, what is unique about humans is that individuals show varying degrees of asymmetry *and* populations show a bias to a particular side, while in other animals individuals show varying degrees of asymmetry but populations are less likely to be biased to a particular side. Since the best evidence in the dyslexic brain implicates strength or degree (rather than direction) of asymmetry, animal studies are an appropriate source of data.

For instance, we found that the size of the primary visual cortex of the rat varies with respect to asymmetry of this structure in the same manner as the planum temporale, i.e., the more total visual cortex there is in a brain, the less asymmetric this architectonic area. We have replicated this relationship between degree of asymmetry and total size of an area in every animal study of asymmetry we have carried out. Also, as with the human planum temporale, in the rat reduction of the cortex, only one side contributes to asymmetry.

We also took advantage of the finding of symmetry and asymmetry of the rat visual cortex to look for a relationship between cell packing density of neurons and degree of asymmetry. We wished to answer the question of whether symmetric cases have more neurons, or are neurons in those cases simply larger and more dispersed one from another. We found that the degree of asymmetry did not correlate with side differences in cell packing density, thus suggesting instead that neuronal numbers might be contributing more importantly to asymmetry or lack thereof (Galaburda et al. 1986). We confirmed this impression in subsequent studies using radioactively labeled neurons, and others also have described asymmetry of neuronal numbers (Williams and Rakic 1988). Therefore, we may conclude that symmetric areas, being larger on one side than asymmetric areas, contain more neurons on that side. Extrapolating to the human case, symmetric plana temporale in dyslexics probably have more neurons in the right side, which is therefore larger. Again, if the finding of symmetry addresses the fundamental mechanism of reading disability in at least some dyslexics, then having more neurons is not better.

What is the origin of the excess of neurons in the dyslexic case and in all other symmetric cases? Excess of neurons may arise from over-production or inadequate pruning. Both neuronal production and pruning represent normal events during the development of the brain, including the cortex. We do not understand in mammals the factors that control neuronal production, but they are likely to be mainly genetic. Neuronal pruning, on the other hand, is genetically controlled but also depends to a significant degree on environmental influences, including competition for connections, correction of developmental errors, and functional needs (Cowan et al. 1984). By "environmental" it is not meant that this is merely the postnatal, including the social and psychological, environment, but also the intrauterine environment that includes physiological and pathological chemical fluctuations to which the developing brain is exposed. Moreover, one neural system is apt to be part of the environment of another during development, such that the development and function of one influences the development and function of the other.

Neurons are produced in the developing human brain very early on, when the neural tube is being formed, and in later germinal zones they continue to be produced for the neocortex (including areas later to be involved in linguistic functions) until probably shortly after the middle of pregnancy (Sidman and Rakic 1973). Neuronal production occurs before neurons migrate to their final cortical locations, after which neurons no longer replicate. In rodents, generation of neurons for the neocortex lasts until the second or third postnatal day. Overproduction of neurons would be apt to reflect (probably genetic) signals acting relatively early in gestation. Pruning of neurons probably occurs to a minor degree soon after the first neurons are produced, but the most active developmental pruning takes place after neuronal migration, probably after the first half of pregnancy in humans, and may continue for a few years after birth (see Huttenlocher 1984). Disturbances in neuronal pruning may point to factors acting after the middle of pregnancy and into the early postnatal period. Thus, the answer to whether the excess in neurons postulated for the dyslexic brains represents overproduction or underpruning could get at the timing of the alteration and hence at the most likely causative agents.

Experiments to address directly the question of overproduction versus underpruning in a developing brain to produce symmetry have not been carried out. Given our current knowledge, such experiments are not plausible because asymmetry of cortical regions cannot be measured during the time in which cell production and pruning take place, and, conversely, when it is possible to assess asymmetry, cell production and cell pruning are long past. An indirect look at the problem using neurons radioactively marked at their birth and followed until maturity is possible and has been carried out in our laboratory. Preliminary findings have not demonstrated differences in cell production to account for differences in cell numbers between symmetric and asymmetric areas (unpublished observations), which increases the odds, but does not prove, that the process of creating asymmetry by pruning of neurons is important here. Additional indirect evidence for cell pruning comes from observations in fetal human brains, which show that asymmetries in the sylvian region, including the area of the planum temporale, do not become evident until after the 30th week of gestation (Chi, Dooling, and Gilles 1977). Neuronal production presumably is finished well before that time and instead postmigrational events, including cell pruning, are more active. It is possible, however, that premigrational events such as cell production begin the process of differentiation between symmetry and asymmetry, which is then magnified postmigrationally during cell pruning. Gross anatomical observations such as those of the fetal brain cannot address this possibility.

Symmetric and asymmetric cortical areas differ in the pattern of callosal connections, and this finding also argues against the concept of "bigger or more is better." Symmetric and asymmetric neocortical areas of the rat were assessed for the pattern of callosal connections by the method of silver degeneration, which outlines dying axonal terminals. The corpus callosum was cut, and the degenerating fibers in both hemispheres were noted in architectonic areas for which asymmetry quotients were also evaluated. Thus, it was possible to assess the relationship between degree of asymmetry and pattern of callosal connectivity. The asymmetric cases were found to have a more restricted pattern of callosal connections than the symmetric cases as assessed by optical density measurements and calculations of the percentage of the area that received callosal terminals (Rosen, Sherman, and Galaburda in press). This could mean that interhemispheric communication is greater (more diffuse) in symmetric cases, including dyslexic brains. This increased callosal connectivity may confer on the brain a disadvantage for processing some forms of linguistic information, and, again therefore, more connections may not be better.

In summary, the presence of symmetry of the planum temporale in the brains of dyslexic individuals raises serious doubts about the phrenologic position. At the gross anatomical level these brains have two large plana. Extrapolation from the animal studies shows that the plana, and consequently language areas, may concern excessive neurons and callosal connections. Less secure is the conclusion that the excessive neurons represent interference with the normal process of neuronal pruning that occurs during (mostly) intrauterine brain development, and the additional axonal terminals might likewise represent diminished axonal pruning. What we have not addressed experimentally at this time is whether this interference with cell and axonal pruning, and therefore presumably an interference with the developmental process by which the nervous system is fine-tuned to meet behavioral tasks, represents in dyslexics a genetic anomaly or an environmental influence during the second half of gestation and early postnatal life.

THE MEANING OF CORTICAL ANOMALIES

The brains of five male and two female dyslexics have shown cortical abnormalities of developmental origin. These have been described in detail elsewhere (Galaburda 1988; Galaburda and Kemper 1979; Galaburda et al. 1985; Kaufmann and Galaburda 1989). In summary, they consist of focal areas of disorganization of the cerebral cortex, namely nests of neurons in the molecular layer (the most superficial layer of the cortex), which does not normally have clusters of neurons, and loss of the neat patterned lamination of the surrounding cortex. There is usually a large number of these foci in each brain, varying in severity and location, but usually affecting the inferior frontal regions and perisylvian cortex, with or without direct involvement of the classical language areas. These types of abnormalities are far less frequent and far less numerous at autopsy in neurologically intact individuals, although they are described in a large number of congenital brain abnormalities (see Kaufmann and Galaburda 1989).

From examination of the abnormalities on routine cell stains, it would appear that the most significant finding is the abnormal location of the cell clusters. Neurons arriving at abnormal locations after migration are probably common, but most of these probably are eliminated as errors during normal cortical development. In experimental studies using mutant strains of mice, the whole pattern of cortical lamination may be reversed, with cells normally destined to occupy deep layers being found superficially, and normally superficial cells being found lying deep in the anomalous cortex (Sidman 1968). Nevertheless, these abnormally placed neurons retain their customary connections, and it is felt that the functional properties of the cortex may not be abnormal (Sidman 1968).

In our cases of focal dysplasia seen in the dyslexic brains, however, the situation may be more complex, the hypothesis being that the neurons in question are not only misplaced, but the affected cortex is different in terms of its cellular and connectional architecture, hence its functional architecture as well.

Several strains of immune defective mice develop abnormalities in the brain that appear to be developmental in origin. Two of these strains, the NZB and BXSB mice, develop clusters of neurons in the molecular layer identical to those found in the dyslexic brains, and we have used them to study these abnormalities to a greater depth than is possible in the human brains (Sherman, Galaburda, and Geschwind 1985; Sherman et al. 1989; Sherman, Rosen, and Galaburda 1988). NZB mice, moreover, show learning abnormalities (Spencer and Lal 1983). One of our studies in the NZB mouse has shown that in addition to their being displaced, at least one of the neuron types in the molecular layer clusters is present in excessive numbers (paper in preparation). Assuming that the focal cortical abnormalities, as well as the symmetry described above, play an etiologic role in the learning disability found in the mouse, and by extrapolation in our dyslexic subjects, this would mean that the excessive neurons in this condition may be damaging to the functional integrity of the cortex. In other words, the presence of focal cortical abnormalities with their extra neurons would also go against the phrenologic claim that more is better.

The cellular abnormalities are so focal that it is difficult to show whether they are normally or abnormally connected to other parts of the brain. However, in one case of focal dysplasia of the cerebral cortex of a rat that had undergone a complete section of the corpus callosum, we were able to show that the pattern of callosal connection to the area of abnormality was also abnormal (Rosen, Galaburda, and Sherman 1989). Furthermore, the abnormality consisted of excessive connections to cortical layers that do not ordinarily receive them. We have begun to confirm this finding of excessive callosal connectivity in artificially induced clusters of molecular layer neurons in the rat (Rosen et al. 1989b).

The focal cortical abnormalities in the dyslexic brains are not always located in the standard language areas. In the standard phrenologic model it would be difficult to explain the linguistic anomalies based on the location of the lesions in all cases. However, in view of the above findings of abnormal connections, the location of these lesions may not be entirely relevant, since the altered pattern of organization of the neuronal networks makes it impossible to determine on purely anatomic grounds what and where the language areas really are in the affected brains.

CONCLUSIONS

The two main findings in the brains of individuals with developmental dyslexia are the presence of symmetry of an important language area of the cerebral cortex and focal areas of cortical malformation that sometimes—but not always—affect the classical language areas. On preliminary grounds both findings are accompanied by excesses in numbers of neurons and some connections. The language area in question in the dyslexic cases is larger rather than smaller than those found in the majority of ordinary brains. These findings argue against the phrenologic hypothesis that bigger (or more) is better, and raise the possibility that under some conditions a bigger neural substrate may be detrimental to some cognitive functions. It also suggests that optimal functional capacity may be related to an optimal match between the number of neurons and connections in a neural net involved in a particular behavior, so that too little or too much is deleterious. Excess being the common factor in both the symmetry and the anomaly found in the dyslexic brains raises the possibility that in these individuals there may be a generalized difficulty with developmental pruning of some neuronal substrates, both in normal development and in elimination of developmental errors, interfering with the achievement of optimal matches. It is not known whether this difficulty has a genetic and/or an epigenetic origin. This question is one focus of ongoing investigations.

REFERENCES

Chi, J. G., Dooling, E. C., and Gilles, F. H. 1977. Gyral development of the human brain. *Annals of Neurology* 1:86–93.
Collins, R. L. 1981. A demonstration of an inheritance of the direction of asymmetry that is consistent with the notion that genetic alleles are left-right indifferent. *Behavioral Genetics* 11:596–600.
Cowan, W. M., Fawcett, J. W., O'Leary, D. D. M., and Stanfield, B. B. 1984. Regressive events in neurogenesis. *Science* 225:1258–1265.
Déjérine, J. 1892. Contribution a l'étude anatomo-pathologique et clinique des differents variétés de cecité verbale. *Comptes Rendus des Scéanses de la Société de Biologie* 4:61–90.
Galaburda, A. M. 1988. The pathogenesis of childhood dyslexia. In *Language, Communication, and the Brain,* ed. F. Plum. New York: Raven Press.
Galaburda, A. M., Aboitiz, F., Rosen, G. D., and Sherman, G. F. 1986. Histological asymmetry in the primary visual cortex of the rat: Implications for mechanisms of cerebral asymmetry. *Cortex* 22:151–60.
Galaburda, A. M., Corsiglia, J., Rosen, G. D., and Sherman, G. F. 1987. Planum temporale asymmetry: Reappraisal since Geschwind and Levitsky. *Neuropsychologia* 25:853–68.
Galaburda, A. M., and Kemper, T. L. 1979. Cytoarchitectonic abnormalities in developmental dyslexia; a case study. *Annals of Neurology* 6:94–100.
Galaburda, A. M., LeMay, M., Kemper, T. L., and Geschwind, N. 1978. Right-left asymmetries in the brain. *Science* 199:852–56.
Galaburda, A. M., and Sanides, F. 1980. Cytoarchitectonic organization of the human auditory cortex. *The Journal of Comparative Neurology* 190:597–610.

Galaburda, A. M., Sherman, G. F., Rosen, G. D., Aboitiz, F., and Geschwind, N. 1985. Developmental dyslexia: Four consecutive cases with cortical anomalies. *Annals of Neurology* 18:222–33.

Geschwind, N. 1968. Anatomy and the higher functions of the brain. *Proceedings of the Boston Colloquium for the Philosophy of Science* 4:98–136.

Geschwind, N., and Levitsky, W. 1968. Human brain: Left-right asymmetries in temporal speech region. *Science* 161:186–87.

Haslam, R. H., Dalby, J. T., and Rademaker, A. W. 1981. Cerebral asymmetry in developmental dyslexia. *Archives of Neurology* 38:679–82.

Hier, D. B., LeMay, M., Rosenberger, P. B., and Perlo, V. 1978. Developmental dyslexia: Evidence for a subgroup with reversed cerebral asymmetry. *Archives of Neurology* 35:90–92.

Hinshelwood, J. 1917. *Congenital Word-blindness.* London: Lewis.

Hochberg, F. H., and LeMay, M. 1975. Arteriographic correlates of handedness. *Neurology* 25:218–22.

Huttenlocher, P. R. 1984. Synapse elimination and plasticity in developing human cerebral cortex. *American Journal of Mental Deficiency* 88:488–96.

Jernigan, T. L., Hesselink, J. R., and Tallal, P. 1989. Cerebral morphology on MRI in language/learning impaired children. Presented at the NIH Conference on Learning Disorders, Bethesda, Md., Sept. 7–8, 1989.

Kaufmann, W. E., and Galaburda, A. M. 1989. Cerebrocortical microdysgenesis in neurologically normal subjects: A histopathologic study. *Neurology* 39:238–44.

Lenneberg, E. 1967. *Biological Foundations of Language.* New York: Wiley Press.

Lubs, H. A., Smith, S., Kimberling, W., Pennington, B., Gross-Glenn, K., and Duara, R. 1988. Dyslexia subtypes: Genetics, behavior, and brain imaging. In *Language, Communication and the Brain* ed. F. Plum. New York: Raven Press.

Rosen, G. D., Galaburda, A. M., and Sherman, G. F. 1989. Cerebrocortical microdysgenesis with anomalous callosal connections: A case study in the rat. *International Journal of Neuroscience* 47:237–47.

Rosen, G. D., Humphreys, P., Sherman, G. F., and Galaburda, A. M. 1989b. Connectional anomalies associated with freezing lesions to the neocortex of the newborn rat. *Society for Neuroscience Abstracts* 15:1120.

Rosen, G. D., Sherman, G. F., and Galaburda, A. M. in press. Interhemispheric connections differ between symmetrical and asymmetrical brain regions. *Neuroscience.*

Rosen, G. D., Sherman, G. F., Mehler, C., Emsbo, K., and Galaburda, A. M. 1989a. The effect of developmental neuropathology on neocortical asymmetry in New Zealand Black mice. *The International Journal of Neuroscience* 45:247–54.

Sherman, G. F., Galaburda, A. M., and Geschwind, N. 1985. Cortical anomalies in brains of New Zealand mice: A neuropathologic model of dyslexia. *Proceedings of the National Academy of Sciences (USA)* 82:8072–8074.

Sherman, G. F., Galaburda, A. M., and Geschwind, N. 1985. Cortical anomalies in brains of New Zealand mice: A neuropathologic model of dyslexia. *Proceedings of the National Academy of Sciences (USA)* 82:8072–8074.

Sherman, G. F., Rosen, G. D., and Galaburda, A. M. 1988. Neocortical anomalies in autoimmune mice: A model for the developmental neuropathology seen in the dyslexic brain. *Drug Development Research* 15:307–314.

Sidman, R. L. 1968. Development of interneuronal connections in brains of mutant mice. In *Physiological and Biochemical Aspects of Nervous Integration* ed. F. D. Carlson. Englewood Cliffs, N.J.: Prentice-Hall.

Sidman, R. L., and Rakic, P. 1973. Neuronal migration, with special reference to developing human brain: A review. *Brain Research* 62:1–35.

Spencer, D. G., and Lal, H. 1983. Specific behavioral impairments in association tasks with an autoimmune mouse. *Society for Neuroscience Abstracts* 9:96.

Williams, R. W., and Rakic, P. 1988. Elimination of neurons from the rhesus monkey's lateral geniculate nucleus during development. *The Journal of Comparative Neurology* 272:424–36.

Chapter • 6

Magnetic Resonance Imaging
Its Role in the Developmental Disorders

Pauline A. Filipek and
David N. Kennedy

Our understanding of the developmental learning
and language disorders depends upon correlations between changes
in behavior and associated changes in the structure of the brain. In
adults, most of the current knowledge has been based on correlations
between discrete focal lesions, usually strokes, and the resulting functional deficits (Kertesz 1983; Geschwind and Galaburda 1985; Damasio
and Damasio 1989). This classical approach, however, is less satisfac-
tory in children for several reasons, but primarily because the majority of these developmental disorders in childhood are not associated
with consistent discrete lesions or recognized pathologic processes
(Denckla, LeMay, and Chapman 1985; Filipek, Kennedy, and Caviness
in press). Therefore, for the purposes of this chapter, these *developmental disorders of learning and language* can be considered as being associated with structural anomalies of developmental origin, resulting in

This work was supported in part by NS 24279 and NS 20489 (Drs. Filipek and Ken-
nedy) from the National Institute of Neurologic Disorders and Stroke, and CA 40303 (Dr.
Kennedy) from the National Cancer Institute; National Institutes of Health, Bethesda,
MD.

very subtle changes in the properties of brain size, shape, and geometric configuration. The challenge is to identify those subtle structural changes that are associated with these disorders in the living child (Caviness, Filipek, and Kennedy 1989; Filipek, Kennedy, and Caviness in press).

The ability to address this challenge has been somewhat limited by available technology. Until 15 years ago, neuroimaging modalities produced only indirect measures of brain disease, such as enlargement of the skull or displacement of the fluid-filled ventricular system within the brain (figure 1A). The development of computed tomography (CT) scans revolutionized clinical and research practices by allowing, for the first time, the direct visualization of actual brain tissue (Hershey and Zimmerman 1985) (figure 1B). However, the anatomic resolution of individual brain structures by CT is less than ideal, resulting in relatively imprecise brain-behavior correlations (Caviness, Filipek, and Kennedy 1989). The subsequent development of magnetic resonance imaging

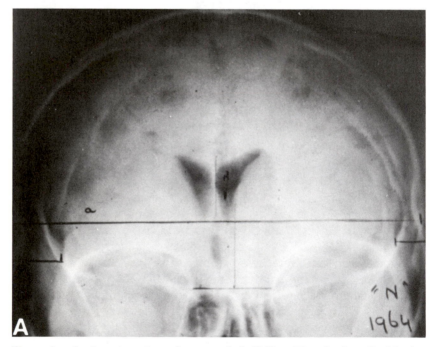

Figure 1. A. Anterior view of a normal skull film. The shadows inside the skull represent the ventricles, which have been filled with air for diagnostic purposes. Note the inability to visualize the actual brain tissue. Photo courtesy of Dr. David Mikulis, Massachusetts General Hospital, Boston, MA. Reprinted with permission from Filipek, P. A., Kennedy, D. N., and Caviness, V. S. In press. In *Handbook of Neuropsychology,* eds. F. Boller and J. Grafman. *Volume 6: Child Neuropsychology,* Topic eds. I. Rapin and S. Segalowitz. Amsterdam: Elsevier Science Publishers.

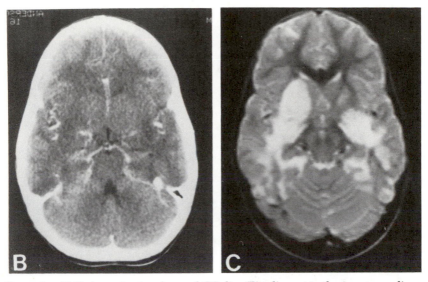

Figure 1.   B-C. A contrast-enhanced CT slice (B) adjacent to the corresponding T$_2$-weighted MRI slice (C) in a child with multiple sclerosis. Note extensive bilateral signal abnormalities predominantly in the white matter on the MRI, which are not visualized on the CT scan. Reprinted with permission from Filipek, P. A. and Blickman, J. G. In press. Neurodiagnostic laboratory procedures: Neuroimaging techniques. In *Pediatric Neurology for the Clinician,* ed. R. B. David. Norwalk, Connecticut: Appleton & Lange.

(MRI) has produced an unprecedented ability to visualize the human brain with clarity comparable to postmortem evaluations (figure 1C) (Consensus Conference 1988; Caviness, Filipek, and Kennedy 1989; Filipek and Blickman in press). With the advent of this technology, we now have the ideal tool to approach the systematic study of developmental disorders with sufficient precision to address the challenge of the developing brain (Filipek, Kennedy, and Caviness in press).

In the following sections, the basic principles of magnetic resonance imaging will be reviewed, followed by a discussion of the applications of MRI in developmental disorders. Some of these applications are still under development; their future implications will be addressed. This technology ultimately will be used to search for the biologic bases for developmental disorders of learning and language.

PRINCIPLES OF MAGNETIC RESONANCE IMAGING (MRI)

The conventional MR imaging system consists of a large magnet of up to 1.5 Tesla magnetic field strength (figure 2A). (1.5 Tesla equals 15 kilogauss field strength, as compared with the earth's magnetic field of ap-

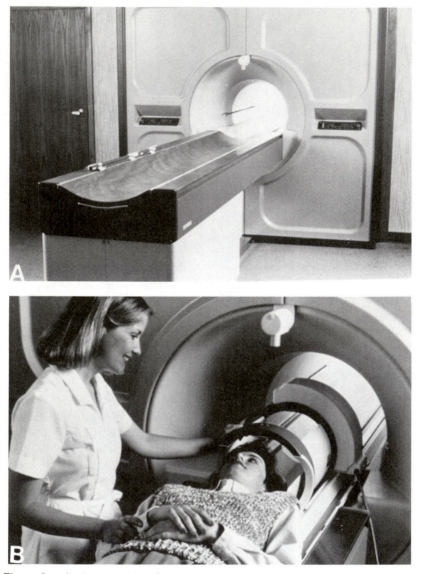

Figure 2.   A. A conventional magnetic resonance imaging system.
B.   A patient resting on the table, as the head coil is moved into position. Note the open "window" that will be positioned in front of the patient's face, and the deep narrow gantry. Both figures courtesy of Siemens Medical Systems, Inc., Iselin, New Jersey. Reprinted with permission from Filipek, P. A. and Blickman, J. G. In press. Neurodiagnostic laboratory procedures: Neuroimaging techniques. In *Pediatric Neurology for the Clinician*, ed. R. B. David. Norwalk, Connecticut: Appleton & Lange.

proximately 5 gauss.) During the scan itself, the patient rests inside a narrow tunnel within the center of the magnet, measuring approximately 8 feet in depth and 30 inches in diameter. For brain imaging, a helmet-like head coil is used, with an open window in front of the face. This coil slides down over the patient's head to the top of the shoulders (figure 2B). Although some adults have severe claustrophobic reactions, most children do not seem to mind the coil or the closeness (Cohen 1986; Filipek and Blickman in press).

Although research is being carried out to develop imaging of elements such as phosphorus or carbon, current MRI technology is limited to hydrogen proton (^{1}H) imaging. Protons are plentiful primarily because of the high water (H_2O) content of the human body. For the purposes of this discussion, these protons can be considered to be randomly oriented in space (figure 3A), although the orientation is not entirely random because of the effects of the earth's magnetic field. When they are subjected to a strong magnetic field such as that inside the scanner, the protons line up with the direction of the field (figure 3B). A radiofrequency (RF) pulse tilts the protons to a characteristic angle (figure 3C), and the protons then give off energy as they return to baseline, much as a gyroscope oscillates from the influence of gravity (figure 3D). This energy is measured and transformed into an image, which can be displayed on a video monitor or filmed for permanent record (Filipek and Blickman in press).

As the protons oscillate back to the baseline, energy is emitted to both adjacent protons and to the environment. This is the basis for the two main parameters measured in MRI, called T_1 and T_2. T_1 measures the energy that is given off to the environment, while T_2 measures the energy that is given off to surrounding protons as they oscillate back to the aligned baseline (Pykett 1982; Cohen 1986). *Pulse sequence* is the term used for an individual MR image acquisition, which can be programmed specifically to demonstrate the differential effects of T_1 or T_2 on brain tissue. These sequences can be made to differ in the frequency of the applied RF pulse, in the angle to which the protons are flipped, and in the time allowed for the protons to relax before another RF pulse is reapplied (Filipek and Blickman in press).

> A *T_1-weighted pulse sequence* produces exquisite detail of the structure of the entire brain, and can be considered as an *"in vivo* anatomic study."
> A *T_2-weighted pulse sequence* is extremely sensitive to strokes, bleeds, and other lesions because of their increased water content. These sequences can be considered as "lesion detectors" (Filipek and Blickman in press) (figure 4).

A clinical MRI scan actually consists of several T_1 and T_2 sequences done consecutively. Each sequence results in a series of serial two-dimensional slices. With MRI, the orientation of the slice can be

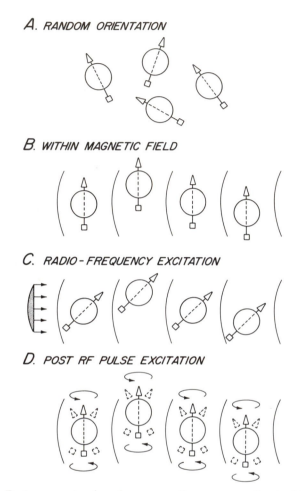

A. RANDOM ORIENTATION

B. WITHIN MAGNETIC FIELD

C. RADIO-FREQUENCY EXCITATION

D. POST RF PULSE EXCITATION

Figure 3.   Basic concepts of nuclear magnetic resonance. See text for description. Figure by Edith Tagrin, Medical Art Resources, Boston, MA. Reprinted with permission from Filipek, P. A. and Blickman, J. G. In press. Neurodiagnostic laboratory procedures: Neuroimaging techniques. In *Pediatric Neurology for the Clinician*, ed. R. B. David. Norwalk, Connecticut: Appleton & Lange.

changed without moving the patient. Therefore, several complementary views of a specific structure or lesion are usually obtained (Filipek and Blickman in press) (figure 5).

CLINICAL USE OF MRI IN THE DEVELOPMENTAL DISORDERS

Magnetic resonance imaging has proved to be an extremely sensitive method for the overall recognition of brain lesions and structural ab-

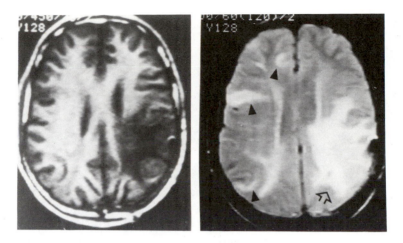

Figure 4.   Representative corresponding slices from a T_1-weighted (left) and a T_2-weighted (right) sequence on a patient with tuberous sclerosis and a tumor, demonstrating the different image characteristics. The T_1-weighted image demonstrates the gray matter-white matter differentiation. The T_2-weighted image is very sensitive to the presence of lesions—the large bright area is the tumor (open arrow). The smaller bright regions (arrowheads) are subcortical hamartomas which are characteristic of tuberous sclerosis. Reprinted with permission from Filipek, P. A., Kennedy, D. N., and Caviness, V. S. In press. In *Handbook of Neuropsychology,* eds. F. Boller and J. Grafman. *Volume 6: Child Neuropsychology,* Topic eds. I. Rapin and S. Segalowitz. Amsterdam: Elsevier Science Publishers.

normalities. Because of the ideal quality of MR images, it was hoped that this new technology would uncover the secrets of the developmental learning and language disorders. However, routine clinical MRI has not yet identified consistent changes associated with these disorders (Denckla, LeMay, and Chapman 1985; Filipek, Kennedy, and Caviness in press).

As mentioned earlier, childhood developmental disorders are usually not associated with lesions, but rather with normal or normal-appearing MRI scans. For example, in the autistic spectrum disorders, although approximately 300 CT or MRI scans have been reported in the literature through 1990, only 15% (45) were clinically read as being abnormal. Of these, only 18 scans demonstrated discrete focal lesions, all of mixed nature and occurring in variable locations in the brain. The other abnormal scans demonstrated nonspecific abnormalities (Filipek, Kennedy, and Caviness in press). In a less severe developmental disability, such as dyslexia, the incidence of abnormal clinical CT or MRI findings is even lower. Of the 255 scans reported in the literature through 1990, less than 7% (15) were felt to be abnormal, demonstrat-

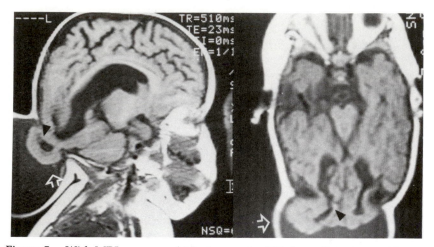

Figure 5. With MRI, one can obtain images in differing orientations without repositioning the patient, which increases the diagnostic utility of the scan. These demonstrate a preoperative sagittal (left) and transaxial (right) MRI views of an occipital encephalocele (a type of spina bifida). Note herniation of occipital lobe into the sac through the defect in the skull (open arrow), including the occipital horns of the lateral ventricles (arrowheads). (TR = 520 msec, TE = 23 msec, slice = 7 mm) Reprinted with permission from Filipek, P. A., and Blickman, J. G. In press. Neurodiagnostic laboratory procedures: Neuroimaging techniques. In *Pediatric Neurology for the Clinician*, ed. R. B. David. Norwalk, Connecticut: Appleton & Lange.

ing rare lesions and a larger proportion of nonspecific findings (Hynd and Semrud-Clikeman 1989; Filipek, Kennedy, and Caviness in press).

The incidence of unanticipated lesions or nonspecific findings in the general pediatric population is currently unknown. Ethical considerations have prevented systematic CT scan studies on normal volunteer children because of the requisite exposure to radiation. Therefore, for control purposes, most CT-based literature reports in the developmental disorders have retrospectively used *scans that appear normal,* as distinct from *scans performed on normal volunteers.* These "control" subjects usually encompass a population with a variety of medical indications for the imaging study, and there is often no control for birth, medical or developmental histories, or academic difficulties (Filipek, Kennedy, and Caviness in press). Several MRI studies are currently in progress which include normal volunteer children and/or children with headaches as control populations, with careful screening for normal histories, neurologic examinations, and academic performance. These subjects constitute the start of a normal MRI-based pediatric data base which may explain the significance of mild anatomic abnormalities (i.e., "nonspecific findings") in the normal childhood population.

Therefore, although MRI is a remarkable technological advance, it does not improve diagnostic capabilities in the *clinical* evaluation of learning, language, or other developmental disorders at this time. So far there have been found no clinically recognized patterns of structural change or lesions that could explain any of these complex behavioral syndromes. However, if we switch from clinical diagnosis to research applications of MRI, we see the potential for identification of anomalies that may enlighten us as to the biological bases for these disorders.

QUANTITATIVE ANALYSES OF CT AND MRI IN DYSLEXIA

The cerebral hemispheres are functionally specialized: the right is predominantly involved with nonverbal visual-spatial functions, while the left is associated with language or verbal functions (Geschwind and Galaburda 1987). The hemispheres are structurally different, with the posterior portion of the "dominant" left hemisphere being wider in 80% of the normal population. In addition, the right far anterior and left far posterior hemispheric tips are more prominent than their counterparts; this prominence is called a *petalia* (Bear et al. 1986).

In developmental dyslexia, less than a dozen neuroimaging studies have been performed on both children and adults (Hier et al. 1978; Leisman and Ashkenazi 1980; Rosenberger and Heir 1980; LeMay 1981; Haslam et al. 1981; Denckla, LeMay, and Chapman 1985; Rumsey et al. 1986; Parkins et al. 1987; Hynd and Semrud-Clikeman 1989; Hynd et al. 1990; Duara et al. in press). Most of the studies have focused on hemispheric asymmetries based on unidimensional linear measurements, such as hemispheric widths measured on individual slices. To generalize, the earlier CT studies in dyslexia reported either symmetric hemispheres (Leisman and Ashkenazi 1980; LeMay 1981) or a reversal of the normal hemispheric asymmetry, with a wider right posterior hemisphere in dyslexics (Heir, Lemay, and Rosenberger 1978; Leisman and Ashkenazi 1980; Rosenberger and Heir 1980; LeMay 1981). Rosenberger and Hier (1980) found a correlation between this reversed asymmetry and lower verbal IQ scores, and Hier, LeMay, and Rosenberger (1978) even proposed this asymmetry as being associated with a high risk for reading disability. Subsequent studies, however, have *not* verified these structural differences in dyslexia using either CT or MRI (Haslam et al. 1981; Parkins et al. 1987; Hynd et al. 1990).

Two additional groups have examined other brain regions, both using unidimensional linear measurements on MRI. Duara et al. (in press) have suggested that both structural and sex differences exist in male and female dyslexics. They reported narrower widths of the *corpus callosum* (the structure connecting the two hemispheres), which may have implications for unusual interhemispheric circuitry in this learning disability. Hynd et al. (1990) reported shorter lengths of the *language areas* of dyslexic brains when compared with controls. In addition, these dyslexic subjects demonstrated a reversal of the expected (left longer than right) asymmetry in the posterior temporal region that includes the planum temporale.

This summary of the few existing neuroimaging reports in dyslexia includes both CT and MRI studies, thereby pooling two imaging methods of differing anatomic resolution. These reports also utilized several different methods of image analysis. The populations have generally been small, with varying diagnostic criteria used to identify the dyslexic subjects. These factors may collectively contribute to the somewhat inconsistent results, and these findings should therefore be considered as *suggestive of* potential structural differences in dyslexia as recognized by CT and MRI (Filipek, Kennedy, and Caviness in press).

Galaburda (1988) has found heterotopias (representing abnormally located collections of cerebral cortex) in postmortem studies on dyslexic subjects. These microscopic abnormalities have been too small to be consistently identified by MRI, which provides spatial resolution of approximately 1 mm (i.e., each picture element, or pixel, in the MRI slice is 1 mm by 1 mm). It also should be understood that the planum temporale, as measured postmortem by Galaburda (1984, 1988), represents solely the bidimensional *surface area* of visualized cortex on the superior surface of the temporal lobe. On conventional MRI slices, it is very difficult to define clearly the borders of this relatively small region as viewed within any given imaging plane for subsequent linear or area measurements (Steinmetz et al. 1989). Head position variability and differences in presenting plane of section (coronal *versus* sagittal) further compound this difficulty. Therefore, measurement of the "planum" on MRI lends itself to potentially high variability across studies, particularly if the pooled parameters include lengths, areas, and volumes (Filipek, Kennedy, and Caviness in press).

MRI-BASED MORPHOMETRY

Rationale

Because of its high anatomic resolution, MRI permits one, for the first time, to perform "patho-anatomic studies" in the living child. This advance now permits the *in vivo* search for those variabilities or anomalies that must be subtle, but may be associated with the causes for these developmental disorders of learning and language. This technological milestone has opened the field for researchers to begin looking for those "needles in the haystacks" in otherwise normal or normal-appearing MRI scans. For the first time, we can now attempt to answer questions pertaining to the structural brain differences that might account for differences in functional abilities in the living child (Filipek, Kennedy, and Caviness in press).

Most researchers in this field recognize that better quantitative methods are necessary to identify the subtle structural changes in the brain as seen by MRI. Unidimensional measures such as hemispheric widths on single slices can be expected to be relatively insensitive to structural changes in the three-dimensional brain. However, these measures have nonetheless identified potentially significant variations in many of these disorders, which can be viewed as the "tip of the iceberg" in our understanding of the developing brain (Caviness, Filipek, and Kennedy 1989; Filipek, Kennedy, and Caviness in press). To increase the sensitivity of MRI-based investigations, a more encompassing view of the *three-dimensional brain* must be undertaken. This approach tests the hypotheses that developmental disorders are associated with subtle abnormalities in the volume (*versus* width or length), two- and three-dimensional shape (*versus* symmetry of linear widths), and geometric configuration of the brain. The field of *morphometry* addresses the measurement of these parameters (Filipek et al. 1989; Caviness, Filipek, and Kennedy 1989; Filipek, Kennedy, and Caviness in press).

Many disease processes produce an increase or decrease of the volume of structures or regions of the brain. For instance, cerebral edema after head injury results in brain enlargement, while the degenerative disorders cause regional or diffuse shrinkage. On this basis, it can be extrapolated that anomalous development may also produce alterations in the volumes of brain structures or functional regions (Filipek, Kennedy, and Caviness in press). However, it has been estimated that the volume of a structure or lesion must differ by as much as 30% to 40% before the change can be visually recognized without measurement. Therefore, routine clinical readings may not identify significant volume changes. This premise has been supported by our preliminary brain tumor analyses, where volumetric changes of up to 50% were not recognized on clinical review (Filipek, Kennedy, and Caviness 1989).

In contrast, the shape and/or three-dimensional topology of the brain may prove to be the more sensitive indices of its fundamental organization. Variations in brain shape may ultimately provide more information than variations in brain size (Galaburda 1984; Geschwind and Galaburda 1985; see also Chapter 5, this volume). For instance, differences in overall brain size among *normal* adults of all ages and races have been shown to have no functional consequence (Gould 1981). In addition, processes occurring early *in utero* may produce subtle changes in the three-dimensional geometric topology of the brain without concurrent volume or shape differences. It is unknown whether distortions exist in the relative proportions of structures, and if they do, whether these distortions may be associated with specific behavioral disorders. Any potential geometric differences might cause or reflect alteration or disruption of circuits in the developing brain (Filipek, Kennedy, and Caviness in press).

Computerized Method of Morphometric Analysis

With this rationale in mind, the domain of morphometry as applied to MRI can now be further explored. The following sections will outline the method that has been developed for MRI-based morphometric analysis of volume, shape, and geometric configuration of the brain. Subsequently, the initial applications performed in pilot studies to date will be reviewed.

Three-dimensional MRI scans. Conventional two-dimensional MRI scans consist of consecutive thick slices, usually 5 to 7.5 mm, with an interslice gap that can vary from 25% to 100% of the slice thickness. For instance, a "5 mm skip 2.5 mm" scan consists of 5 mm slices with a 2.5 mm gap in-between (equal to 50% of slice thickness). It is important to realize that the portion of the brain that occurs within the gaps *is not imaged*. In addition, these routine MRI scans often do not image the entire brain, but rather end within an inch of so of the edges. Any morphometric analyses performed on these scans either interpolate through these gaps or consist only of area measurements on single slices. Either approach results in a high error because of these factors (Filipek et al. 1989; Filipek, Kennedy, and Caviness in press).

An additional factor consists of "volume averaging," which refers to the fact that each two dimensional slice represents the average of all the signal intensities through the depth of the slice, rather than just the surface. The thicker the slice, the greater are the effects of volume averaging on the analysis. For example, because of volume averaging, morphometric analysis on three contiguous 2.5 mm slices will be more representative of the underlying anatomy than it would on a single 7.5 mm slice through the same region. Therefore, the rate of error for morphometric analysis will be lower with a thinner slice (Filipek et al. 1989; Filipek, Kennedy, and Caviness in press).

To diminish these causes of error, an MRI scan to be used as the basis for morphometric analysis must consist of thin contiguous slices that cover the entire brain, while providing detailed anatomic resolution of gray and white matter structures, all within a reasonable imaging time of less than 15 minutes. Most conventional MRI scanners cannot routinely produce such a T_1-weighted sequence (for anatomic resolution), although this availability is increasing. A three-dimensional T_1-weighted sequence has been specifically adapted for use as the basis for subsequent morphometric analysis. This sequence meets the requirements mentioned above, producing 60 contiguous 3 mm slices to cover the whole brain in less than 15 minutes imaging time, with high resolution of grey and white matter structures (figure 6) (Filipek et al. 1989).

Image segmentation. The core operation of this MRI-based method for morphometric analysis requires that the entire brain be segmented into its anatomic components. Volumetric, shape, and geometric analyses are subsequently performed on these segmented regions (figure 7). At the outset of this endeavor in 1985, computer-assisted hand-drawn outlines were performed, taking approximately four hours to process each individual slice of the scan, with an inherently high rate of error. Because of this time factor, it was not feasible to apply this morphometric method to large statistically-mandated popu-

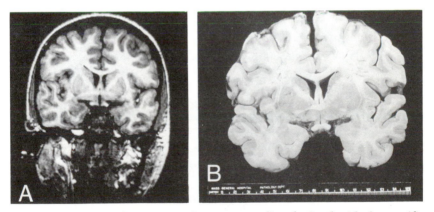

Figure 6. Representative magnetic resonance slice obtained with the specifically-adapted three-dimensional T_1-weighted spoiled gradient echo pulse sequence (A) shown for comparison next to a corresponding slice from a human autopsy specimen (B). Note the improved anatomic resolution of the MRI scan, which demonstrates virtually all the structures seen pathologically. Compare this with the lower resolution of the CT scan shown in Figure 1B. Pathologic specimen courtesy of Dr. David Lewis, Massachusetts General Hospital, Boston, MA. Reprinted with permission from Filipek, P. A., Kennedy, D. N., and Caviness, V. S. In press. In *Handbook of Neuropsychology,* eds. F. Boller and J. Grafman. *Volume 6: Child Neuropsychology,* Topic eds. I. Rapin and S. Segalowitz. Amsterdam: Elsevier Science Publishers.

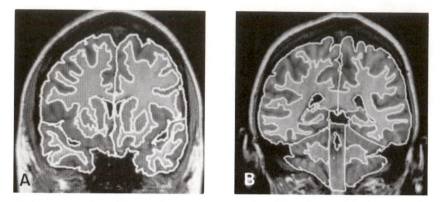

Figure 7.   Representative magnetic resonance slices after application of the morphometric algorithms, demonstrating the border-defining contours of the anatomical structures. The morphometric calculations of volume, shape, and geometric localization are subsequently performed on these contours.
A. Anterior coronal slice demonstrating the segmented cerebral cortex, white matter, basal ganglia, and ventricles.
B. Posterior coronal slice demonstrating the cerebral cortex, white matter, ventricles, cerebellum and brainstem. Reprinted with permission from Filipek, P. A. et al. 1989. MRI-based brain morphometry: Development and application to normal subjects. *Annals of Neurology* 25:61–67.

lations. Semi-automated computer algorithms have subsequently been developed for image segmentation to produce full morphometric analyses of the brain and its substructures with far greater efficiency (Kennedy 1986; Kennedy, Filipek, and Caviness 1989; Filipek et al. 1989).

An *intensity contour-mapping* algorithm was created to produce continuous outlines at structural borders based on the signal intensity of the pixels. This computerized technique improves the accuracy and efficiency of the analyses relative to the original manual method, although it still involves a significant amount of interaction and subjectivity. To decrease this investigator interaction, subjectivity, and error, an objective mathematical edge-detection approach has been taken, using a Sobel edge-enhancement operator (Pratt 1978). This *automated image segmentation algorithm* automatically creates a contour, requires minimal interaction, and markedly decreases the time required for the analysis. It uses the outline from the previous slice as the initial estimate for the current outline and self-adjusts this estimate on the current slice. It then proceeds to the next adjacent slice, repeats the entire process, and essentially "walks through" all 60 slices of the scan. When fully operational, the aim is to "walk" the contours of all structures from plane to plane simultaneously. This will require interaction only to add new structures as they appear, or to correct errors before they propagate through the entire scan (Kennedy, Filipek, and Caviness 1987, 1989; Filipek et al. 1989).

Positional normalization and geometric topology. Because head position within the scan varies between subjects, comparison of anatomic structures in the original "native" orientation can be difficult, increasing the inherent error of the method (Filipek, Kennedy, and Caviness 1989). A homogeneous three-dimensional coordinate transformation is performed on each native MRI and its segmentation outlines (Filipek, Kennedy, and Caviness 1988 in press) based on standardized anatomic reference points (Talairach and Tournoux 1988) (figure 8). The native MRI scans and outlines are then both resliced to

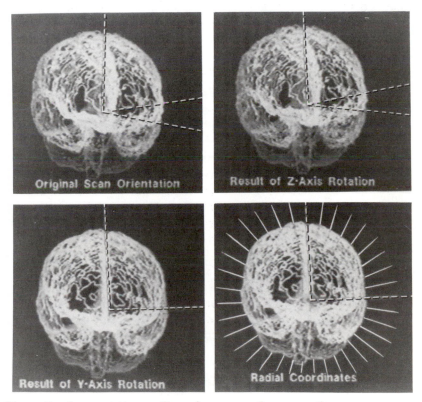

Figure 8. Segmentation outlines from an entire magnetic resonance scan, with superimposed X, Y, and Z axes. The sections demonstrate each step of the positional normalization process, using the three-dimensional coordinate system. The final section demonstrates the spherical radial coordinates used for the geometric localization analyses. Reprinted with permission from Filipek, P. A., Kennedy, D. N., and Caviness, V. S. In press. In *Handbook of Neuropsychology*, eds. F. Boller and J. Grafman. *Volume 6: Child Neuropsychology*, Topic eds. I. Rapin and S. Segalowitz. Amsterdam: Elsevier Science Publishers.

create almost identical positionally normalized MRI scans and outlines (Filipek, Kennedy, and Caviness 1989). This post-processing technique eliminates the need for a special positional protocol during the scan itself, which is particularly advantageous when working with children. It also compensates for any patient movement between the individual T_1 and T_2 sequences, and normalizes the orientation of scans obtained across a large study cohort (Filipek, Kennedy, and Caviness 1989, in press).

The resulting normalized spherical coordinate system is the basis for subsequent analysis of geometric topology (Filipek, Kennedy, and Caviness 1988). Any identified region of interest can be characterized in terms of its position within this system, resulting in measures of radial and angular extent and the center of mass coordinates. This co-ordinate system also permits the evaluation of three-dimensional shape (Sacks et al. 1990), further described below, and allows correlations between MRI and functional imaging modalities, such as positron emission tomography (PET) (Alpert et al. 1990).

Shape analysis. A method for shape characterization of the brain and its structures has been developed using Fourier spatial frequency distribution analysis (Filipek et al. 1988; Kennedy et al. 1988; Kennedy, Filipek, and Caviness 1990). This technique evaluates the complexity of brain shape by evaluating up to twenty spatial frequency harmonics, each representing the number of lobes within the structure (figure 9). For example, a simple circle has a harmonic of zero, while a figure-of-eight has a harmonic of two. Separate evaluation is performed for the horizontal-vertical and diagonal directions to quantify the contribution of each harmonic to the structural shape. The result is a set of "A" and "B" coefficients, respectively, for each harmonic. Although shape analysis has been used extensively in other sciences, for example geology (Erlich and Weinberg 1970), this approach has not previously been extended to brain science. Using this technique, the two- and three-dimensional shape of the brain and its structures now can be quantified for the first time for comparison across large study populations.

APPLICATIONS OF THIS MRI-BASED METHOD OF MORPHOMETRY

Volumetric Determinations

Normal adults. This morphometric method was applied to MRI scans obtained on seven adult volunteers with normal head circumferences and neurologic examinations (Filipek et al. 1989). The volumes of whole brain and substructures were calculated, and the results are presented in table I. These are the first reported estimates of absolute

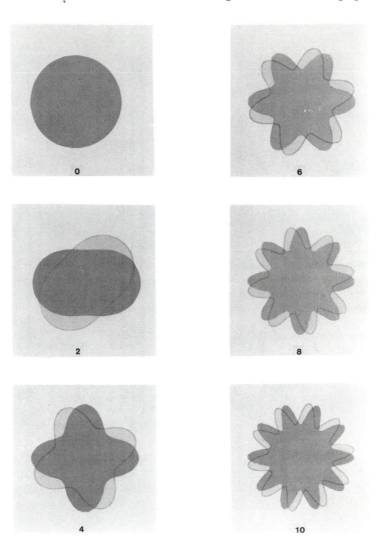

Figure 9.   Artist's rendition of the Fourier harmonics and coefficients used in two-dimensional shape analysis of the brain. The number of the Fourier harmonic represents the number of lobes in the structure, with higher numbers for more complex figures (see numbers under each figure). A simple circle has a harmonic of zero. The A coefficient (darker figures) measures the horizontal and vertical shape. The B coefficient (lighter figures) measures the diagonal shape. Figure by Edith Tagrin, Medical Art Resources, Boston, MA. Reprinted with permission from Filipek, P. A., Kennedy, D. N., and Caviness, V. S. In press. In *Handbook of Neuropsychology*, eds. F. Boller and J. Grafman. *Volume 6: Child Neuropsychology*, Topic eds. I. Rapin and S. Segalowitz. Amsterdam: Elsevier Science Publishers.

Table I.   MRI-Based Morphometric Volumes in Normal Subjects

Anatomical Region	MRI-Based Volume in CM³ (N = 7)	Normal Fresh Volume in CM³ (N = 31)
Whole brain	1,343.4 ± 126.9	1,370.6 ± 139.6
Cerebral hemispheres	1,181.9 ± 119.7	1,197.6 ± 125.6
Cerebral cortex	762.7 ± 53.2	772.0 ± NA*
Cerebral white matter	400.6 ± 72.1	NA
Ventricular system	15.8 ± 4.9	14.4 ± 6.3
Caudate	6.7 ± 1.7	NA
Putamen	8.5 ± 1.2	NA
Globus pallidus	2.1 ± 0.2	NA
Diencephalon	19.2 ± 2.4	NA
Cerebellum	140.9 ± 17.1	142.0 ± 16.0
Brainstem	20.9 ± 3.2	NA

Values expressed as the mean ± standard deviation.

The mean age at death for the postmortem series was 63.5 years (Wessely 1970; Paul 1971).

*N = 1 (Kretschman et al. 1979).

MRI = magnetic resonance imaging; NA = not available.

Reprinted with permission from: Filipek, P. A. et al. 1989. MRI-based brain morphometry: development and application to normal subjects. *Annals of Neurology* 25:61–67.

volumes based on an MRI-based method of morphometry, and are concordant with previously published volumes of normal fresh (unfixed) brains obtained postmortem (Wessely 1970; Paul 1971; Kretschman et al. 1979). Although notable variability is apparent for each structure, the MRI-based standard deviations are similar to those found for the unfixed pathologic specimens. Multiple factors may contribute to this range of standard deviations, including the biologic variation of human neuroanatomy. Because of the small subject number, it was not feasible to evaluate sex-related differences. Until more subjects can be evaluated, it is unclear whether these volumetric calculations are representative of the normal population as a whole.

Volumetric measures in two siblings.   Two normal right-handed siblings, an 18-year-old male and a 16-year-old female, volunteered to participate in our MRI study (Filipek et al. 1988). Each attained at least an 85th percentile in academic achievement tests and never had evidence for learning disabilities. The brains of these siblings both demonstrated a reversal of the normal cerebral asymmetry, with a left frontal and right occipital predominance. The volumes of each region were also concordant for every measure in the two sibling brains (table II). These results indicate that the role of genetic influences in the determination of brain form holds great promise, especially with identical *versus* fraternal twin comparisons (Caviness, Filipek, and Kennedy

Table II. Regional Hemispheric Volumes in Two Siblings

Anatomic Segment		Sibling Volumes Male	Female	Control Mean Volumes (± standard deviation)
Hemispheres	Right	676.4	629.8	613.4 ± 80.0
	Left	666.9	620.7	616.4 ± 72.2
Precallosal	Right	79.7	70.8	84.3 ± 4.9
	Left	96.0	88.3	91.4 ± 14.8
Pericallosal	Right	341.7	271.1	263.0 ± 59.4
	Left	334.6	271.1	267.2 ± 51.6
Anterior superior	Right	71.1	63.6	71.0 ± 19.3
	Left	72.3	72.8	71.2 ± 20.1
Anterior inferior	Right	38.1	30.1	36.1 ± 15.2
	Left	35.0	33.9	36.0 ± 12.1
Posterior superior	Right	106.1	104.2	87.7 ± 13.4
	Left	103.9	105.4	93.1 ± 7.9
Posterior inferior	Right	39.1	32.9	40.4 ± 6.1
	Left	40.1	31.3	39.3 ± 5.1
Anterior temporal	Right	23.1	20.2	29.8 ± 7.0
	Left	35.4	35.7	32.3 ± 9.5
Posterior temporal	Right	67.0	69.6	57.5 ± 7.4
	Left	63.7	72.3	52.2 ± 8.8
Retrocallosal	Right	164.9	198.1	178.8 ± 9.7
	Left	137.2	153.3	173.4 ± 17.6

1989). Further studies are ongoing to evaluate other members of this family.

Developmental language disorders. The National Institutes of Health is currently supporting an ongoing multicenter longitudinal research project, headed by Dr. Isabelle Rapin, to characterize developmental language disorders and autism in 600 children over an eight year period. Verbal auditory agnosia (VAA) is one type of developmental language disorder, and is characterized by the selective inability to understand spoken language despite preserved hearing, inner language, and the preserved ability to read and write (Rapin and Allen 1988). VAA has an almost exact counterpart in adult pure word deafness, which is usually caused by bilateral strokes in the posterior temporal (language) regions. Children with VAA can understand gestures, can learn sign language and, with special instruction, can learn to read and write. The major difference from the adult syndrome is that these children are mute or severely dysfluent. Adults with pure word deafness probably remain fluent after strokes due to the fact that language becomes overlearned, while preschoolers with VAA have not yet acquired sufficient, if any, language (Rapin and Allen 1988).

There are very few pathologic correlates for any of the developmental language disorders. In the single reported autopsy on a child with VAA, bilateral cystic lesions were found in the posterior temporal regions (Landau, Goldstein, and Kleffner 1960). Lou, Henricksen, and Bruhn (1984) performed a cerebral blood flow study in one child with VAA and noted decreased blood flow at rest in the posterior perisylvian language regions bilaterally. With verbal activation studies, the expected increase in blood flow to the language areas did not occur.

As the initial MRI pilot study for this multicenter project, we examined four adolescents with VAA (Filipek et al. 1987). Two of the MRI scans were clinically read as normal, while the third scan demonstrated nonspecific cerebral atrophy. The fourth scan demonstrated a focal lesion in the left posterior temporal region. This was consistent with a very large subcortical heterotopia (relative to the dyslexia studies mentioned earlier), representing an abnormally located collection of cerebral cortex (figure 10).

When the volume of each whole cerebral hemisphere was calculated, there were no differences between the VAA subjects and the controls. To improve the sensitivity of the volumetric measures, an arbitrary method was devised to segment the hemispheres into smaller regions which might be more closely analogous to known functional areas, such as the perisylvian regions for language function. Each hemisphere was therefore segmented into precallosal, anterior and posterior pericallosal, and retrocallosal regions, based on the location of the corpus callosum in the MRI scan. Again, no significant differences were found between the VAA and control subjects. Each pericallosal region was further segmented into superior, inferior, and tem-

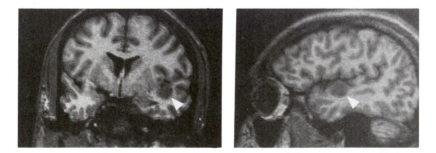

Figure 10.   Coronal (left) and sagittal (right) MRI slices demonstrating left superior temporal heterotopia (arrow) in an adolescent with verbal auditory agnosia. A CT scan did not demonstrate any abnormalities. (TR = 40 msec, TE = 15 msec, slice = 3.1 mm). Reprinted with permission from Filipek, P. A., and Blickman, J. G. In press. Neurodiagnostic laboratory procedures: Neuroimaging techniques. In *Pediatric Neurology for the Clinician*, ed. R. B. David. Norwalk, Connecticut: Appleton & Lange.

poral subdivisions, to more closely define the known language areas (figure 11).

When each of these subdivisions was evaluated, a significant difference was found between the VAA subjects and the controls. A focal volumetric decrease was found in the posterior temporal segments of the VAA brains, significant to $p < .05$ for the right posterior temporal region, and showing a trend for the left posterior temporal region, with $p < .20$. The posterior temporal regions are those affected in acquired adult word deafness and in the single VAA autopsy. These findings support the hypothesis that subtle morphologic anomalies may be identified by morphometric analysis and will follow known functional neuroanatomy.

Error analysis. We applied the volumetric method to MRI scans of a standardized "phantom" containing 1000 cc ($\pm$ 5 cc) of water (Fil-

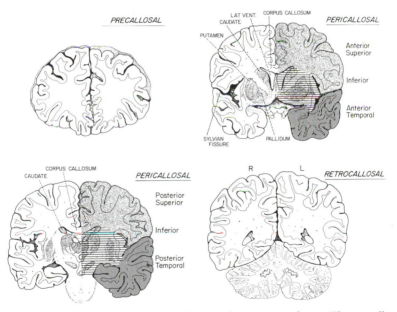

Figure 11. "Callosal" regions used for morphometric analyses. The *precallosal and retrocallosal* regions are those anterior and posterior coronal slices, respectively, that do not visualize the corpus callosum. The *anterior and posterior pericallosal* regions are defined by the appearance of the third ventricle. The superior, inferior, and temporal pericallosal regions are defined by hand-drawn borders. Figure by Edith Tagrin, Medical Art Resources, Boston, MA. Reprinted with permission from Filipek, P. A., Kennedy, D. N., and Caviness, V. S. In press. In *Handbook of Neuropsychology,* eds. F. Boller and J. Grafman. *Volume 6: Child Neuropsychology,* Topic eds. I. Rapin and S. Segalowitz. Amsterdam: Elsevier Science Publishers.

ipek et al. 1989). Including error from the actual acquisition of the MRI scan itself, the aggregate error of the morphometric method was found to range from 4.5% to 9.6% with the value dependent upon slice thickness (figure 12). The error for the thin slices we routinely use is 5.2%, as compared with the error of postmortem morphometric analyses, which can range over 20% (Williams, Ferrante, and Caviness 1978). Sources of MRI-based error potentially include inhomogeneities in the magnet itself, the pulse sequences, and slice thickness, as well as the morphometric analysis. The sources of error from the magnet itself cannot be analyzed individually at this time for independent contribution to the overall aggregate error.

Shape Analysis

Two-dimensional Fourier shape analysis was performed on the posterior cerebral hemispheres of the two siblings mentioned in the preceding section (Filipek et al. 1988). Because a cerebral hemisphere is essentially a bilobed organ, one would expect a difference in hemispheric shape to be demonstrated in the second Fourier harmonic. There was a difference in the right second harmonic for the sibling

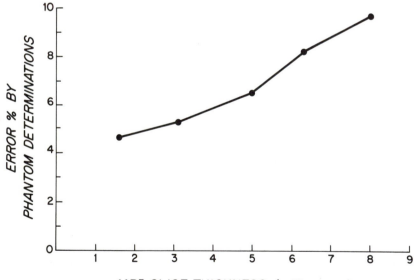

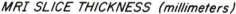

Figure 12.   Percent error of the MRI-based method of morphometry as a function of MRI slice thickness, based on phantom measurements. At 3 mm, the error is approximately 5%. Reprinted with permission from Filipek, P. A. et al. 1989. MRI-based brain morphometry: development and application to normal subjects. *Annals of Neurology* 25:61–67.

brains, demonstrating that their right hemispheres are wider and diagonally narrower than the controls, while the left hemispheric shape is the same. These measures reach significance for the B2 coefficient, with $p < .05$ in this small cohort (figure 13). These findings not only support the reversal of normal hemispheric asymmetry but also quantify brain shape for the first time. This shape analysis is being applied to the developmental language disorder cohort and to the normal controls in an attempt to determine the shape characteristics of the brain in developmental disorders.

Cerebral Cortical Parcellation

Although the anatomic subdivision method described earlier produces hemispheric segments that include those regions pertinent to language function and improves the analytic sensitivity of the method, these "callosal" segments often incorporate numerous functional regions or cross functional boundaries. With the development of a three-dimensional coordinate system for geometric localization, we have considered additional methods for analyzing specific functional cortical-subcortical regions. We are developing a system of cerebral cortical

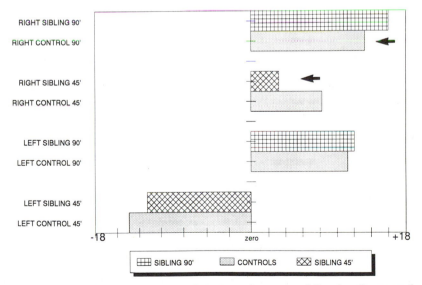

Figure 13.   Graphic presentation of the two-dimensional Fourier shape analysis performed on the MRI scans of two siblings with a reversal of the normal hemispheric asymmetry. Because a hemisphere is essentially a bi-lobed structure, the 2nd Fourier harmonic would be most sensitive to hemispheric shape differences. The analysis quantifies the wider and diagonally narrower (arrows) right hemispheres in the siblings, when compared with the controls.

parcellation (Kennedy et al. 1989) which has been adapted from the functional summary by Mesulam (1985) and the Talairach Atlas (Talairach and Tournoux 1988). This parcellation is coarse and anatomically approximate, but it subdivides the cerebral hemispheres into regions dictated by principles of cerebral organization and accommodates the concept of cerebral anatomy that is traditional to structural-functional correlation studies (Filipek, Kennedy, and Caviness in press).

The cortical functional subdivisions of the human brain may be identified by their correspondence to relatively constant fissures and gyri on the surface of the brain. To aid in the three-dimensional visualization of the brain, we have developed a method for surface rendering the segmentation contours (Kennedy et al. 1989). This produces a three-dimensional presentation of any given brain imaged by our MRI method, on which the principle surface landmarks may be easily identified. This technique will define those cerebral cortical regions hypothesized to be affected on a functional basis in any given disorder, and will improve the sensitivity of the morphometric analyses (Filipek, Kennedy, and Caviness in press).

MRI-Based Blood Volume/Blood Flow Studies

Blood flow and blood volume within the brain have been useful experimental measures to evaluate the physiologic functioning of the brain, both at rest and with activation studies. For instance, Posner et al. (1988) used positron emission tomography (PET) to observe the brain processes involved during single word activation studies. They found increased cerebral blood flow to the occipital lobes (the portion of the brain that "sees") when the subjects were visually presented with nouns to read. When the words were presented in auditory form, blood flow increased in the left temporal-parietal region (the known language areas).

Until very recently, any *in vivo* measure of blood flow or blood volume was limited to PET or single photon emission computed tomography (SPECT). Both methods require the administration of a radioactive isotope. PET scanning additionally requires the presence of a nearby cyclotron for the generation of its short-lived isotopes (Reivich and Alavi 1985). In addition, the higher radiation risk from the isotopes, and the potential for invasive intra-arterial access severely limits the use of these functional imaging techniques in children. For these reasons, PET or SPECT scanning is not feasible for large functional imaging studies.

Dr. Bruce Rosen and his colleagues (1989) at Massachusetts General Hospital have developed a method for blood flow and blood volume measurements using MRI in a relatively noninvasive technique.

Instead of requiring a radioactive isotope and intra-arterial access, this method uses the routine MRI contrast agent called gadolinium-DTPA. This method takes advantage of the MRI signal diminution in the brain as a bolus of gadolinium-DTPA passes through the brain capillary system. The time course of the signal change is related to the capillary blood volume and blood flow rates.

Since the first passage of this bolus through the brain is completed within approximately 20 seconds after the intravenous injection in the normal individual, extremely rapid imaging techniques must be employed in order to characterize the changes in signal intensity over time. These rapid imaging techniques are currently implemented on the *Instascan* (Advanced NMR, Woburn, MA) MRI system that acquires each single MR slice in *less than 1 second,* as compared with routine MRI studies averaging 5 to 15 minutes. This rapid imaging permits the real-time visualization of the passage of the gadolinium through the brain in a second-by-second time frame. An actual movie loop can then be made of the passage of each bolus of gadolinium through the brain. Based on the differential signal intensities of each pixel (picture element) of the image as a function of time, *blood volume* can be calculated across the brain. Current endeavors are focused on the development of *blood flow* techniques based on this method, which is more complicated, but which holds promise to provide significant functional information, similar to that obtained with the more invasive PET methods.

Although the anatomic resolution of the *Instascan* is less than that obtained with the specifically-adapted MRI scans mentioned earlier (Filipek et al. 1989), the combination of these two techniques for MRI-based blood flow and three-dimensional T_1-weighted MRI scans for morphometric studies may well permit both structural and functional evaluations during a single MRI scanning session. Because gadolinium-DTPA is approved for use in children, and only a single "needle-stick" is required, structural-functional correlations may now become feasible in children with developmental disorders.

CONCLUSIONS

In conclusion, there is presently little indication for the routine use of MRI in the diagnosis of the developmental learning or language disorders. However, methods based on MRI are currently being developed for *in vivo* anatomic studies to correlate changes in brain structure with altered function, with particular emphasis on the developmental disorders of childhood. Future endeavors include large statistically mandated populations of children with these disorders, as well as the initiation of a normal childhood "brain" data base for comparison studies.

REFERENCES

Alpert, N. M., Bradshaw, J. F., Kennedy, D. N., and Correia, J. A. 1990. The principle axis transformation–A method for image registration. *Journal of Nuclear Medicine* 31:1717–1722.

Bear, D., Schiff, D., Saver, J., Greenberg, M., and Freeman, R. 1986. Quantitative analysis of cerebral asymmetries. Fronto-occipital correlation, sexual dimorphism and association with handedness. *Archives of Neurology* 43:598–603.

Caviness, V. S., Filipek, P. A., and Kennedy, D. N. 1989. Magnetic resonance technology in human brain science: A blueprint for a program based upon morphometry. *Brain and Development* 11:1–13.

Cohen, M. D. 1986. *Pediatric Magnetic Resonance Imaging.* Philadelphia: W. B. Saunders Company.

Consensus Conference. 1988. Magnetic resonance imaging. *Journal of the American Medical Association* 259:2132–2138.

Damasio, H., and Damasio, A. R. 1989. *Lesion Analysis in Neuropsychology.* New York: Oxford University Press.

Denckla, M., LeMay, M., and Chapman, C. 1985. Few CT scan abnormalities found even in neurologically impaired learning disabled children. *Journal of Learning Disabilities* 18:132–35.

Duara, R., Kushch, A., Gross-Glenn, K., Jallad, B. J., Pascal, S., Barker, W. W., Loewenstein, D., and Lubs, H. A. In press. Neuroanatomical features of dyslexia on MR scans. *Archives of Neurology.*

Erlich, R., and Weinberg, B. 1970. An exact method for characterizing grain shape. *Journal of Sedimentation Petrology* 40:205–212.

Filipek, P. A., and Blickman, J. G. In press. Neurodiagnostic laboratory procedures: Neuroimaging techniques. In *Pediatric Neurology for the Clinician,* ed. R. B. David. Norwalk, CT: Appleton & Lange.

Filipek, P. A., Kennedy, D. N., and Caviness, V. S. 1988. A method of morphometric analysis of the human brain based upon magnetic resonance imaging. *Annals of Neurology* 24:356.

Filipek, P. A., Kennedy, D. N., and Caviness, V. S. 1989. Morphometric analysis of central nervous system neoplasms. *Annals of Neurology* 26:461.

Filipek, P. A., Kennedy, D. N., and Caviness, V. S. In press. Neuroimaging in child neuropsychology. In *Handbook of Neuropsychology,* eds. F. Boller and J. Grafman. *Volume 6: Child Neuropsychology,* Topic eds. I. Rapin and S. Segalowitz. Amsterdam: Elsevier Science Publishers.

Filipek, P. A., Kennedy, D. N., Caviness, V. S., Klein, S., and Rapin, I. 1987. *In vivo* MRI-based volumetric brain analysis in subjects with verbal auditory agnosia. *Annals of Neurology* 22:410.

Filipek, P. A., Kennedy, D. N., Caviness, V. S., Rossnick, S. L., Spraggins, T. A., and Starewicz, P. M. 1989. MRI-based brain morphometry: Development and application to normal subjects. *Annals of Neurology* 25:61–67.

Filipek, P. A., Kennedy, D. N., Kennedy, S. K., and Caviness, V. S. 1988. Shape analysis of the brain of two siblings based upon magnetic resonance imaging. *Annals of Neurology* 24:355.

Galaburda, A. M. 1984. Anatomical asymmetries. In *Cerebral Dominance,* eds. N. Geschwind and A. M. Galaburda. Cambridge, MA: Harvard University Press.

Galaburda, A. M. 1988. The pathogenesis of childhood dyslexia. In *Language, Communication and the Brain,* ed. F. Plum. New York: Raven Press.

Geschwind, N., and Galaburda, A. M. 1985. Cerebral lateralization. Biological mechanisms, associations, and pathology: A hypothesis and a program for research. *Archives of Neurology* 42:428–59, 521–52, 634–54.

Geschwind, N., and Galaburda, A. M. 1987. *Cerebral Lateralization.* Cambridge, MA: The MIT Press.

Gould, S. J. 1981. *The Mismeasure of Man.* New York: W. W. Norton.

Haslam, R., Dalby, J. T., Johns, R., and Rademaker, A. 1981. Cerebral asymmetry in developmental dyslexia. *Archives of Neurology* 38:679–82.

Hershey, B. L., and Zimmerman, R. A. 1985. Pediatric brain computed tomography. *Pediatric Clinics of North America* 32:1477–1508.

Hier, D., LeMay, M., Rosenberger, P. B., and Perlo, V. P. 1978. Developmental dyslexia: Evidence for a subgroup with a reversal of cerebral asymmetry. *Archives of Neurology* 35:90–2.

Hynd, G., and Semrud-Clikeman, M. 1989. Dyslexia and brain morphology. *Psychological Bulletin* 106:447–82.

Hynd, G., Semrud-Clikeman, M., Lorys, A., Novey, E., and Eliopulos, D. 1990. Brain morphology in developmental dyslexia and attention deficit disorder/hyperactivity. *Archives of Neurology* 47:919–26.

Kennedy, D. N. 1986. A system for three-dimensional analysis of magnetic resonance images. Masters thesis. Department of Nuclear Engineering, Massachusetts Institute of Technology, Cambridge, MA.

Kennedy, D. N., Filipek, P. A., and Caviness, V. S. 1987. Semi-automated image segmentation in multi-slice magnetic resonance brain images. *Proceedings of the Society of Magnetic Resonance in Medicine* 6:378.

Kennedy, D. N., Filipek, P. A., and Caviness, V. S. 1989. Anatomic segmentation and volumetric calculations in nuclear magnetic resonance imaging. *Institute of Electrical and Electronic Engineers Transactions on Medical Imaging* 8:1–7.

Kennedy, D. N., Kennedy, S. K., Filipek, P. A., and Caviness, V. S. 1988. Morphometric characterization of brain shape by Fourier analysis. *Proceedings of the Society of Magnetic Resonance in Medicine* 7:993.

Kennedy, D. N., Filipek, P. A., and Caviness, V. S. 1990. Fourier shape analysis of anatomic structures. In *Recent Advances in Fourier Analysis and its Applications,* eds. J. S. Byrnes and J. L. Byrnes. Dordrecht, The Netherlands: Kluwer Academic Publishers.

Kennedy, D. N., Rowell, D., Filipek, P. A., and Caviness, V. S. 1989. Neural system segmentation of three-dimensional magnetic resonance brain images. *Proceedings of the Society of Magnetic Resonance in Medicine* 8:983.

Kertesz, A. 1983. *Localization in Neuropsychology.* New York: Academic Press.

Kretschmann, H. J., Schleicher, A., Grottschreiber, J. F., and Kullman, W. 1979. The Yakovlev collection: A pilot study of its suitability for the morphometric documentation of the human brain. *Journal of Neurological Science* 43:111–26.

Landau, W., Goldstein, R., and Kleffner, F. 1960. Congenital aphasia: A clinicopathologic study. *Neurology* 10:915–21.

Leisman, G., and Ashkenazi, M. 1980. Aetiological factors in dyslexia: IV. Cerebral hemispheres are functionally equivalent. *Neuroscience* 11:157–64.

LeMay, M. 1981. Are there radiological changes in the brains of individuals with dyslexia? *Bulletin of The Orton Society* 31:135–41.

Lou, H. C., Henricksen, L., and Bruhn, P. 1984. Focal cerebral hypoperfusion in children with dysphasia and/or attention deficit disorder. *Archives of Neurology* 41:825–29.

Mesulam, M-M. 1985. Patterns in behavioral neuroanatomy: Association areas, the limbic system, and hemispheric specialization. In *Principles of Behavioral Neurology,* ed. M-M. Mesulam. Philadelphia: F. A. Davis Company.

Parkins, R., Roberts, R. J., Reinarz, S. J., and Varney, N. R. 1987. CT asymmetries in adult developmental dyslexics. *Journal of Clinical and Experimental Neuropsychology* 9:41.

Paul, F. 1971. Biometrische Analyse der Frischvolumina der Grosshirnrinde und des Prosencephalon von 31 menschlichen, adulten Gehirnen. *Zeitschrift fur Anatomie und Entwicklungsgeschichte* 133:325–68.

Posner, M. I., Petersen, S. E., Fox, P. T., and Raichle, M. E. 1988. Localization of cognitive operations in the human brain. *Science* 240:1627–1631.

Pratt, W. K. 1978. *Digital Image Processing.* New York: John Wiley & Sons.

Pykett, I. L. 1982. NMR imaging in medicine. *Scientific American* 246:78–88.

Rapin, I., and Allen, D. A. 1988. Syndromes in developmental dysphasia and adult aphasia. In *Language, Communication and the Brain,* ed. F. Plum. New York: Raven Press.

Reivich, M., and Alavi, A. 1985. *Positron Emission Tomography.* New York: Alan R. Liss, Inc.

Rosen, B. R., Belliveau, J. W., and Chien, D. 1989. Profusion imaging by nuclear magnetic resonance. *Magnetic Resonance Quarterly* 5:263–81.

Rosenberger, P., and Hier, D. 1980. Cerebral asymmetry and verbal intellectual deficits. *Annals of Neurology* 8:300–304.

Rumsey, J. M., Dorwart, R., Vermess, M., Denckla, M., Kruesi, M., and Rapoport, J. 1986. Magnetic resonance imaging of brain anatomy in severe developmental dyslexia. *Archives of Neurology* 43:1045–1046.

Sacks, J., Kennedy, D. N., Filipek, P. A., and Caviness, V. S. 1990. MRI-based three-dimensional analysis of shape. *Proceedings of the Society of Magnetic Resonance in Medicine* 9:100.

Steinmetz, H., Rademacher, J., Huang, Y., Hefter, H., Zilles, K., Thron, A., and Freund, H. J. 1989. Cerebral asymmetry: MR planimetry of the human planum temporale. *Journal of Computer Assisted Tomography* 13:996–1005.

Talairach, J., and Tournoux, P. 1988. *Co-Planar Stereotaxic Atlas of the Human Brain.* New York: Thieme Medical Publishers, Inc.

Wessely, W. 1970. Biometrische Analyse der Frischvolumina des Rhombencephalon, des Cerebellum und der Ventrikel von 31 adulten menschlichen Gehirnen. *Journal fur Hirnforschung* 12:11–28.

Williams, R. S., Ferrante, R. J., and Caviness, V. S. 1978. The Golgi-rapid method in clinical neuropathology. I. Morphologic consequences of suboptimal fixation. *Journal of Neuropathology and Experimental Neurology* 37:13–33.

Discussion

DUANE: First, I want to make a comment, Herb, on your reference to the handedness issue. The practice I have now in Arizona is a peculiar one. It may reflect the neurologist who has it. We work with three groups of patients. One is a group of patients we have called behavioral neurology, that includes learning disorders and a population of patients referred by psychiatrists where the possibility of some organicity in the psychiatric syndrome is raised. The second group is a group of individuals who are dystonics: focal or generalized. The third is a more general group of neurologic patients. All of those patients fill out an Edinburgh laterality questionnaire and the laterality quotient is generated. An observation we have made with a pool of 100 patients in each group suggests that the dystonics are not only right handed, but strongly right handed when the movement disorder begins in adult life. In the behavioral group, both learning disorder and psychiatric referral patients, the Laterality Quotient (LQ) scores for right handedness are not only lower than the dystonics, but lower in comparison with the general population of neurologic patients. It may be useful to the work that you and others do to go beyond the question of right or left handedness and to specify the degree of handedness. You may also wish to specify whether or not there is crossed lateralization for eye and hand use. Have you ever considered this?

LUBS: We have used the same score. I just didn't have time to present that. I suspect we are talking about apples, oranges, and apricots here. Our assumption is that many of the children, who were brain damaged at birth or had some other environmental early life insult and who ended up with a learning disability, are probably those who have the increased frequency of left handedness, at least within our apple sample, if you will. The laterality scores are just fine. So I am guessing this is an ascertainment bias and we are looking at a different population. In terms of the crossed lateralization, it is a good suggestion and again, we at least now have the ability with the MacIntosh computer to cross check all of the parameters. We are very anxious to put in all of our brain parameters, the PET findings, and see what correlates with what, what runs with what within a family; but there is so much we haven't been able to do.

DUANE: Herb, you have said that this autosomal dominant group of yours should have an equal frequency of male and female dyslexics. It wasn't clear from your presentation that you had an equal representation in your groups. Yet John DeFries' observations, and he just had an article in the *Journal of Learning Disabilities*, showed that there was a gender effect. Who is right?

LUBS: Well, that is easy to answer, partially with solid data and partially by inference. Look at the audience out here. I was trying to count while Albert was talking, but his talk was so interesting, I only got about a quarter of the way through the audience. The sex ratio is 7.2:1 (females to males) in this audience. This is an ascertainment bias. You are here because you are interested in this. You are working in this field. That plays, I think, a very large part in all of this. Plus the apples, oranges, and apricots again. We do have slightly, not excessly, more males than females in our study and in Shelly Smith's original study. However, this ratio is not statistically significant from the expected 50/50. That, I think is ascertainment bias and probably because, as I said, males, if they get bored in school and can't do the work, are going to get into trouble. Teachers are going to recognize them. They are going to get sent for special evaluations. I think they get recognized more often. I suspect they also are more severe and therefore get recognized more often just on that basis alone.

Then there must be another group of people, perhaps brain damaged at birth, in whom there probably is a sex ratio that is in favor of more males than females. There is no evidence of a sex-linked form of dyslexia that I know of. That, too, is easy to rule out because once you have transmission from a father to a son, it cannot be on the X chromosome because the son would be a daughter. And, I know of no such family. I don't think that we, and everybody, could have missed it. It is very unlikely that there is a sex-linked form of dyslexia. These other biases probably all add up to the gender difference. It would be interesting to get the others' thoughts.

DUANE: Why are the risk factors that you found, John, not equivalent between mothers and fathers?

DEFRIES: Well, the risk issue gets to the possible application of what is referred to as a polygenic threshhold model. I am not sure you really want to get into the details of that today, but I would like to say just a word about prevalence rates in terms of a possible gender-ratio difference. In a paper that is currently in press, Susan Vogel makes a very important point. She says there is a real difference between referred populations of reading-disabled children versus research identified samples. That is consistent with my experience.

In the Colorado Family Reading Study that I talked about first this morning, which is a referred sample, the gender ratio is about 3.5:1 (male to female). A very typical gender ratio. On the other hand, the gender ratio in our twin study is a research identified sample, which is close to 1:1.

Is there a gender ratio that deviates from 1:1? My guess is that it probably does a little bit, but I don't think the gender ratio is anywhere close to 3.5:1. My recollection was that in your initial study, Herb, you did find an excess of males. But in the relatives you found that the gender ratio was much closer to 1:1.

LUBS: Again, that is presumably an ascertainment bias. The males are more affected, the families are more concerned, so those are the ones that join the studies. In any analysis of autosomal dominant inheritance, you throw out the proband because he biases the results in the direction of being affected.

DUANE: When you use the word "severity," are you talking about how severely impaired the reading ability is, or are you talking about other manifestations?

LUBS: Next year when we have a follow-up symposium, maybe we can answer that. We are trying to put all of our reading scores together in different ways to see if we can come up with some sort of index of severity. We don't have one yet. This is just clinical impression that there are more males and more severely affected males, even within these families. However, I can't quantify it.

DEFRIES: In some of my recent analyses with my colleagues, Dick Olson and Bruce Pennington, if you look at the gender ratio as a function of severity, you do find that the ratio increases. In other words, relatively more males than females are at the more extreme end of the distribution. That makes me think that there really is some difference in the actual gender ratio. That is, it is not truly 1:1. I think there is some excess of males, but it depends a little bit upon how severely one selects in terms of the samples and the way in which they are ascertained.

GALABURDA: I agree. I have another related comment pertaining to three studies. I am going to cite Paula Tallal's Society of Neuroscience abstract showing that in fact if you look at dyslexia that is passed through the maternal line (and there are those), as opposed to those that are passed through the paternal line, the number of girls born to those families is diminished. Also, in David Urion's subpopulation of patients of Irish descent who have learning disability, auto-immune disease, left handedness, and premature graying of the hair there are also fewer girls born in the families. The third group is Bob Lahita's population of lupus mothers. They gave birth to dyslexic boys, very commonly, up to 45%. And there were fewer girls born to those mothers. So one of the reasons for less dyslexia in girls may have something to do with the fact that fewer girls are born in families who are susceptible. Of course you have to consider the possibility that they are not born because they are really so severely affected that they die soon after conception.

Now if one looks at our autopsy cases, in fact the most severe brain changes that we have seen in any of the brains have been in females. If you look at Martha Denckla's studies, I think she has been quite clear that when dyslexia is diagnosed in females, it tends to be more severe and more atypical. So we have a lot of confusing issues here that need to be resolved.

DUANE: Let me add one other point, and that is, how generalizable are your anatomic findings with regard to other conditions, without using the word *disorder*, other conditions of the human spirit? What other diagnoses have you encountered in the population of patients that you have examined? For instance, for those working in education or in psychology, there is a large population of under or erratic achievers, who have what is called attention deficit hyperactivity disorder [ADHD]. How many, if any, of the population you have examined, have that trait? There is an overabundance of psychiatric diagnoses among those with school underachievement. Is there a higher prevalence of another condition that would suggest that there may be co-existent other conditions that might be linked causally?

GALABURDA: No one is too anxious to take that one.

LUBS: We do have the hyperactivity scale that teachers fill in that has been used in all of our studies. And, in a few people, this [ADHD] is present. This does complicate the study. If there is too much ADHD or it appears to be the predominant problem, we don't study those families. We omit those in the name of simplifying things and keeping a clearer study sample. There are a few people who are isolated within a family who have had such a problem. We note it. We have it. We will look at it, but if ADHD is a big problem, we exclude them.

DEFRIES: We don't have any really good clinical diagnoses in terms of attention deficit disorder. We are currently using a questionnaire, the Diagnostic Interview for Children and Adolescents (DICA), to try to get a handle on it. The prevalence is much higher than we had thought, something like 30%.

LUBS: Clinical investigation is still an art and the definition unfortunately becomes very much like that of politics. It is the art of the possible. I think it would be fascinating to use this same approach that we have made with reading on families with pure attention deficit, and nothing else. I think there are several cases clinically of such children. Some who persist with this through life and some who get better after puberty. I would love to know the pedigrees of these families. I think it is possible there is a subgroup that is autosomal dominantly inherited. That investigation would be possible using the same linkage techniques that have been used in studies of dyslexia. We would like to be able to do that one of these days, when we have nothing else to do.

DUANE: What arrangements have been made by either of you to see that any of the subjects in your studies, should they succumb, would have their central nervous systems examined by Al Galaburda?

DEFRIES: We have done nothing. It is tough in the case of school age twins or singletons to say, "By the way we know of this other interesting study that is being conducted where we need brains for autopsies." I recognize the import of the question, and I am not trying to be facetious about it. I have tried to think my way through it as to how one should really handle this ethically. I must confess I haven't really resolved the issue.

LUBS: We have said, if you can survive our study, you are going to live forever! So it is not going to be a problem! But, you are asking us this, of course, for a pointed reason. We should be thinking of this and obviously we should be trying. We have thought about this in several families where there are older family members. We still haven't quite had the courage to tackle it, but we should and thank you for asking it.

DUANE: I think it is quite possible to introduce brain donation as a consideration as part of the materials given to a family participating in the study without being offensive. Indeed, you might be surprised at how positively this is received by families. Obviously not by the children. Also if there should be a tragedy and the child is lost, the sense that there might be something learned as a consequence often times gives parents a sense of consolation. Al and various members of The Orton Dyslexia Society could advise us on a sensitive, appropriate approach.

DUANE: Bennett, I notice in your series of students you indicated that you would exclude students with seizures who are on medication for the seizure disorder. What about the instance of a student who would have had a history of a single nocturnal seizure and who was not kept on medication? Would that student be eliminated from your investigation?

SHAYWITZ: Yes, we do exclude students with a history of a seizure or epilepsy.

DUANE: The reason I raised that particular point—as Al will remember, in the first case that he and Tom Kemper reported in 1979— that student at the age of 16 had a single nocturnal seizure. Our experience has been that a number of the students with learning problems we see may have an occasional seizure. They don't have epilepsy in the sense of recurrent seizures but an occasional febrile or nocturnal seizure seems not to be rare in the broad spectrum of students who have academic problems.

Al, I wonder if you could comment on the possible connection with epilepsy. I have always thought that epilepsy and especially temporal lobe epilepsy and dyslexia may be rather more closely related than we had thought. I wonder if you or others find similar ectopias in the brains of epileptic patients?

GALABURDA: That first patient had clinical epilepsy. It was very mild but it needed to be treated. Our first dyslexic female patient probably had temporal lobe epilepsy although it was never diagnosed. She fit the clinical description of a temporal lobe epileptic. And it really seems quite fair to say that some of the pathology that we know about epilepsy is very similar to the pathology that we have described in dyslexic individuals. There have been several studies describing cortical heterotopias in the molecular layer of epileptic patients similar to those in our dyslexic patients. The same sorts of errors in wiring that might lead to processing difficulties could also lead to epilepsy, although the story is far from clear.

I want to emphasize that I, and I suspect most of us here on the panel, would not want to link epilepsy to either a learning disability or attention disorder. I think, historically, the medical community did a good job in convincing educators that children who looked inattentive may have petit mal epilepsy. And I can tell you that we get innumerable children referred each year by educators who think that the children have petit mal epilepsy when in fact they have a learning disorder or an attention disorder. I don't want people to go away thinking that there is a relationship between epilepsy and learning and attention disorders. The two may occur in the same child but I think it is quite rare. Epidemiologic studies of children with learning disabilities or with attention disorders don't show an increased prevalence of seizures.

DUANE: On the other hand, however, within a referral population, the incidence of epileptiform discharges in the EEG of such patients seems inordinately high. I have wondered whether the changes that Al has described in these dyslexics might be seen in a broader percentage of the population who are non-dyslexic but who have other behavioral syndromes.

Frank, the work that you did with PET at UCI showed functional symmetry with respect to glucose metabolism. Is there a way in which you can correlate that activity with Al's speculation and observation that the total number of neurons is increased in the dyslexic nervous system? That is, can you compare the average nervous system versus the dyslexic nervous system with respect to symmetry, and is there increased cortical neuronal activity?

WOOD: It's easy to make a superficial correlation. I guess the best thing I ought to do is tell you one or two of the things that give us pause before rushing out to endorse that. I mean I agree with it. I would like to endorse it and be done, but there are one or two annoying facts that stand in the way. The main one, it seems to me, would be this implication that the increased cell population, let's say, in a dyslexic brain, would be associated with less specificity either of the cross callosal connections or even of gray matter areas in a cortical mosaic type of model. And yet the scans that we see seem to have a lot of punctate activity in the dyslexic brain. I would have thought that you would see a big red blush across a dyslexic brain if all it had was more neurons. Instead, one sees lots of hot spots that are too hot, maybe, but this is not uniform. So it is complicated.

Furthermore, there is always difficulty in correlating morbid anatomy with functional anatomy. What Al sees under the microscope may not be visualized as functional activity because those neurons may not be active.

The PET scan measures energy consumption by a variety of ways. It does not really address the issue of higher dysfunction. Let's say that it is easy to conceive in evolutionary terms that some parts of the brain in fact use less energy to do the same job. So the fact that something lights up in the PET doesn't mean necessarily that it is participating in the proper way for doing something. You could have more neurons but they may not be doing much and consequently generate less activity. You could have a few neurons trying very hard to participate, thus using up a lot of energy which lights up the PET. Frank Duffy's studies, particularly those kids who recovered, showed that a lot of the brain does in fact participate in these children in an electrical way, which is another way of looking at participation. So in the end we have to put together three types of observations: anatomy, electrophysiology, and energy consumption to try to make some sense out of this.

DUANE: I agree, and that comment introduces a question raised from the audience about brain electrical activity mapping (BEAM) or computer assisted EEG. I think that it gives us an additional dimension by which we can make comparisons but which are not identical to the morbid anatomy or the functional anatomy as measured by, say, cerebral blood flow.

Pauline, perhaps you are aware of the work being done at Ohio State University's Department of Psychiatry and Psychology? They are doing some three dimensional brain reconstructions through MRI scans. They have had the provocative notion of trying to combine that three dimensional imaging with power spectral analyses from the electroencephalogram. Mike Torello is doing that project. Is there any chance that you and your coworkers in Boston may try to also provide that projection on the cortex so that you may visualize in 3-D the surface electrical activity?

FILIPEK: Yes, it is something that I did not mention today because I am not an electrophysiologist. The language disorder program project that I referred to will use MRI and a three dimensional surface rendering in conjunction with Herbert Vaughn's sophisticated three dimensional electrophysiology at Albert Einstein University. So we will be able to correlate the 3-D EEG that he has been getting with these children's MRIs. The children are actually located in Cleveland, New York, and Boston and their MRI tapes get sent to me.

DUANE: A question raised from the audience is, do any of you believe that there is any relationship between any of the learning disabilities, dyslexia or others, with migraine? Herb, how about those families that you are working with? Do they have a lot of migraine?

LUBS: We have not had a particular history of it. Bruce Pennington might want to comment on that.

DUANE: There has been an association among those with migraine having a higher rate of arterial venous malformation or AVM. And as Al has shown there are some dyslexic individuals who had symptomatic AVMs in childhood. They tend to be in the left hemisphere as I recall. Is that correct Al?

GALABURDA: Yes, but I would say that that's probably a very small proportion of all dyslexics. At this point we don't know what is the clinical significance. I wouldn't worry about it in clinical terms. There are other issues, however. Migraine is very common and what's called migraine in clinical populations is even more common even though it's not migraine. In the end, the numbers of subjects you have to study to be able to determine a significant link is enormous. I don't think any of the studies were of that size. Certainly among our eight dyslexics who came to autopsy, none of them had migraine. We all know thousands of migraine patients without dyslexia. But obviously that's not the answer to the question. There may be an interesting interaction through left-handedness for instance, for we do know that there is a relationship between left-handedness and migraine.

DUANE: Pauline, you made a reference to MRIs not being helpful in childhood autism. Yet Terry Jernigan and Eric Courchesne and their colleagues have published some data that suggests there may be an anatomic correlation in the posterior fossa with autism. What is your view?

FILIPEK: No. I'm saying that first of all Terry and Eric measure and quantitate the posterior fossa as well. I don't think that we know enough about the posterior fossa in general to be able to say if routinely, in all autistic children, there is a decreased area of the cerebellar vermis as seen on a sagittal MRI scan. When I say that it is not clinically useful I mean the visual threshold is somewhere between 40 and 50% reduction before you can consistently see a change in volume. This is what a clinical radiologist routinely looks for before applying a clinical interpretation. If we have colleagues from Johns Hopkins or the University of Pittsburgh, they may be able to answer the question better than I. Both centers have sought to replicate these findings and so far have been unable to do so on their own sample of autistic children. It's at least fair to say that most autistic children do not have measurable, quantifiable hypoplasia of the cerebellar vermis, though without question, some do.

DUANE: Let me get back to something that has been, I think, an interesting observation by more than one group that has presented today. That is the refutation of the previously held notion that dyslexic behavior is more prevalent in males as opposed to females. The question that I would ask is why did the population studied in England by Michael Rutter and his team show a male preponderance? Similarly, Isabelle Liberman's investigation, which looked at the bottom third readers in a second-grade classroom, also showed a male preponderance. However, I would agree with the observation made that behavioral disturbance may be more prevalent in males, i.e., ADD, and thus may be referred on the basis of their activity level. But both of the above-mentioned were population studies. What is the reality regarding gender and dyslexia?

LUBS: We've talked a lot about male/female differences. If you look at many reading tests you'll see a difference in the distribution between males and females. However, the distribution is tighter in females and wider in males. There are more bright males and more dumb males. Thus, if you look at the bottom third of a distribution on many tests, males are likely to come out worse I suspect.

SHAYWITZ: Let me quote some of the data, actually from my wife's longitudinal study, which look at an epidemiologic sample of children who had been followed up since kindergarten and who are now in sixth grade. There was a sample that was recruited in a random fashion from around the state and represented a random selection of Connecticut kindergartners in a particular year. What she's found is that using a school-based definition of a reading disability there are many more boys, perhaps three or four to one, depending upon the grade that is examined. However, using a research definition, a discrepancy definition for example, the numbers of boys and girls who would be identified as having a reading disability are identical. So that suggests that, in fact, referral bias is a major factor in the presumed increased prevalence of reading disability in boys. Indeed there are other data in older literature to support this finding, although not from an epidemiologic sample. The data again suggest that referral bias is the major influence on the so-called increased prevalence of reading disabled boys over girls.

GALABURDA: We've come around full circle now. If you believe the studies of families where dyslexia is prevalent, and not all dyslexics obviously, but at least those that are passed through the maternal line (work by Paula Tallal and David Urion), there are fewer girls in those families. Now we are finding out that under certain forms of definition of the disorder there is an equal number of male and female dyslexics. That means that dyslexic girls are much more vulnerable to the disorder, because there are fewer of them. We really have to settle this one, otherwise we have opposite answers in the same conference.

It seems to me that what you need to do is to decide which definition to use, as depending upon which definition is employed you will arrive at different answers. Thus we need agreement, or one must say, given a particular definition of reading disability, particular consequences will follow. Given one particular definition, one of those consequences might be that there won't be an increased prevalence of boys over girls. Given another definition there might be. I think that it is important to know how you are defining the term so that you know what are the consequences. My guess is that we can only agree on the fact that given a particular definition, there will be a particular consequence.

Just a comment, also, on Paula Tallal's data, which upset a lot of things. I've looked at them and thought about them. They make no sense but there they are. Maternally passed dyslexia occurs in families with more boys than girls. So one has to come back to the old saw, which is, "The hardest things to explain are those which are not so." I suspect this is a bias that the missing children just don't make any sense. Somehow there has got to be a bias that even the most rigorous of us cannot as yet find. I do not concur with those studies that don't agree with respect to the gender issue. If two or three studies make roughly the same observation using a scientific definition, there may be equal numbers of affected girls and boys. Alternately, the girls don't get referred because people don't care as much about their reading achievement. In either instance, should dyslexic behavior be as common in girls as it is in boys, our observations are still important. It may mean that females are more vulnerable, which would be consistent with the immune hypothesis. It could be that hypothesis which would explain the reduction in females through immune diseases. These are more common in females and as a consequence females may be more vulnerable to their adverse effect. This offers a tentative hypothesis which is capable of being tested. It could be that the female fetuses are spontaneously aborted, balancing the equation. A study of spontaneous abortion might provide an answer in this regard.

LUBS: The sex ratio is only 1.06 at conception. I don't think it would explain all of that.

GALABURDA: That's exactly my point, if you assume roughly equal sex rates at conception, you have to assume a greater rate of spontaneous abortions after conception among girls. That's an empirical prediction and should be testable, I would think.

LUBS: As far as I know, we know much more about the sex ratio at birth than at conception. That would be a very hard thing to do. It's a scientific challenge because even in animals there are very few reliable markers for the Y-chromosome genes. It's getting better, but it's hard to do at conception. However, at birth the sex ratio in humans is slightly in favor of boys. The boys begin to die in the first decade and in the end by the time we get to be eighty there are virtually only women around. But the fact is that if there are fewer girls born in those families, that means even something unusual is happening because there should be more boys in most families.

DUANE: One of our audience members wonders if the sex differences in reading disorders is of a developmental bias. That is, this person accepts that girls learn to read younger. So, if we study first graders or perhaps beyond that, we will see more boys but by the seventh grade the bias would disappear. Is there data to support that?

LUBS: Well I don't know. I think that is a good point. There do seem to be different trajectories of the development of cognitive skills between boys and girls. Whether those trajectories would intersect at some point in development such that you would get equal rates of disability at one point and not at another is an interesting idea.

WOOD: At least the data that we've seen through third grade beginning as early as first grade indicates that, using a definition that we would consider to be fairly rigorous, there were no sex differences. Whether by the time the children get to be seventh graders the trend would change is not known. We will be able to look at them in fifth grade very shortly.

DUANE: We have a couple of questions that are somewhat similar. One asks whether language remediation induces structural brain changes. The other asks if there is any evidence of a change in any of the biological measures as a result of successful treatment of dyslexics? I'll add, do those of you who have the Dyslexia Institutes and are following your patients longitudinally look for changes in these measures and correlate them with clinical improvement?

WOOD: It is a clear result of our data that some of Mrs. Orton's students got to be essentially normal readers who had been measurably dyslexic, i.e., two standard deviations below the mean as children. These compensated adults show the same blood flow redistribution as persisting dyslexics show. That would suggest that something really happened to them with respect to their treatment which was quite interesting because it did *not* change the basic redistribution of function that they presumably were born with, but in some other way, bypassed their handicap. I would say that would be the usual case. However, I suspect that there are some situations in which intervention actually changes not just the function but the structure. If pressed, I could maybe give a couple anecdotal examples of it, but without ruling out the possibility that you could change even the structure somewhat. I would say that for the most part, the redistribution of function in the brain that takes place persists, and that the intervention accomplishes its desired results despite not changing the underlying structure.

DUANE: Is that observation an argument for very early identification even before the emergence of some acquired language skills?

WOOD: To me it is and I invite you all to attend Dr. Felton's presentation which offers further encouraging evidence from our studies about the effects of early identification and remediation.

GALABURDA: As a morphologist, it may sound funny for me to say this, but ultimately the important thing is the function not the structure. Now we want to know about the structure for our own private biological reason, mostly intellectual. It's also important to know that no matter what happens to us, normal or dyslexic alike, the structure of the brain does change and that such changes occur in response to learning and other environmental factors. No doubt the structure is changing. But, the important thing is outcome. In some cases who have remediation they have gotten better and in other cases they have not. So we are not actually measuring the parts of the brain that are making the change. That is, by the way, very common. We don't hit the right place at the right time all the time. We may not even be looking at the right level. In fact, what PET studies may measure, which is metabolic rates and synaptic activity, may not be at a level at which all of this is happening. It may be happening at the level of axonal wiring which is not measured by the PET scan at all.

So the important thing to show in fact is that a particular remediation program, whether it is educational, psychological, or medical, works. The rest is less important. It is interesting but not necessarily important.

DUANE: Herb, I have a question for you because you've got the perspective that few have, looking at three generations and seeing individuals longitudinally or at least at various stages of their own evolution. An occasional clinical observation is that individuals may give you a history that when they were children they struggled in a given academic subject only to improve. But as they mature, and super mature, sometimes those mid-life compensated-for defects become more troublesome for them. So that naming difficulties may occur more readily at the age of 60 (in some of these people) rather than waiting until the age of 70 or 75. Is there any evidence from the longitudinal evaluation of your patients that those difficulties that were prevalent in childhood re-emerge as senescence approaches?

LUBS: We haven't asked about that in our older family members. It would be interesting to go back and do that. So I don't have any data on it. Frank, do you have any?

WOOD: Well, I have only an anecdotal example. You understand our probands are adults usually in their thirties. We study their children, who would be second generation now, but we also study their parents to try and get three generations.

We just ran into a set of parents and we haven't seen but a dozen or so parents of these adults. And this parent sure was strange. He was 55 or 60 years old and he looked for all the world like a well compensated Alzheimer's patient. But his wife said, "You know he's really been that way for a long time and he still is functioning rather well on his job," and so forth. I think this may be something that we will find. I'll just go ahead and predict that we may find more of this outcome than you'd find in an ordinary population. There is an analogy to this in those who follow high functioning autistics or who follow what we call pervasive developmental disorder in children who are essentially high functioning autistics in one way or another, i.e., milder autistics. They also seem to get better by adolescence. Then in later adolescence and adulthood, rather like these dyslexics we're talking about, they seem to start to decline again. So this is not an unfamiliar concept to me.

LUBS: We're talking anecdotally, of course. I've collected large numbers of friends because I am interested in this. So looking at my friends, of which there are half a dozen who are aged 60 and have rather severe dyslexia, they are all sailing along and doing fine. They haven't had any of these troubles so maybe some do but certainly most of the people that I know are doing extremely well.

DUANE: That's the case for at least one of the female dyslexics in Al's project.

GALABURDA: There's a tendency because of what we have learned about Down syndrome which is what I think colors what we know. Down syndrome children develop very slowly and their language acquisition is very slow and impaired. They become old very young. By 15 or 20 years they have senile tangles and plaques in their brains that look very much like Alzheimer's disease. There are a lot of biological clocks that work like that. Women who have their menarche at 15 or 16 as opposed to 12 or 13 tend to stop their periods early. So that things that start late tend to end early biologically speaking, much the same way as if you put a bad carburetor into a car it will go first before anything else. However, I agree that there is very little evidence that in dyslexia that is the case and that it isn't quite your standard disease situation where you have a downgraded system that will break down a little sooner. What we have seen however, and we are trying to collect more cases, is that individuals who have had some learning disability or some very early developmental neurological disturbance develop tumors perhaps more often in those areas. That's a bit frightening if that turns out to be true. It's something that we are looking at. There are several examples in the literature of people who were, let's say, dyslexic and then developed temporal lobe tumors.

DUANE: We have seen three in the last two years since I've been in Scottsdale. They're low grade and probably congenital tumors.

GALABURDA: Low grade anyway. Two of our cases had tumors.

DUANE: Frank, as I recall one of your presentations in the past, your group has tried to identify the dyslexia pure from the dyslexia plus category of June Orton's population. The dyslexia plus are those that also had ADD. Do you care to make any comment about that combined group versus the pure syndrome as to differential outcome?

WOOD: I was trying to escape from doing that but I'll go ahead and do it since you asked. In this group, which divides out into suitable numbers for all three or four subgroups, here's what we found. You have this whole group of people who June Orton saw. We've now seen a total of 144 of them. Some of them are dyslexic and some of them are not. And some of them, by blind scoring of her interviews of their parents, are ADD and some are not. Some are both and some are neither. What we find in the multivariant analysis of those data is rather striking. If you know of a child in her sample, IQ and socioeconomic status in childhood, you can predict their educational outcome and learn nothing more about predicting their educational outcome by knowing that they are dyslexic. That is to say, June Orton's dyslexics had just as many years of formal education after high school or including high school as June Orton's non-dyslexics did, once you equate them for their IQ and their socioeconomic status. The same was not true for attention deficit disorder however.

If you looked at somebody and found that they were ADD as a child, you'd predict an average of two years less formal education than for the non-ADDs. This is regardless of whether they were dyslexic or not. So this is to say that it is attention deficit disorder in that sample that is really associated with long-term underachievement scholastically rather than dyslexia itself. But I have to make a couple of other comments. I don't think that it is proper to describe a pure ADD or a pure dyslexic. That's like saying somebody is a pure boy or pure girl. People are a variety of things usually. Almost always there are several things at once and I am not sure that pure ADD or pure dyslexia is a concept we should accept. Sufficient unto the day is the evil thereof, and if you have a child with dyslexia or ADD or both, they each need treatment and there are appropriate treatments for each of those conditions. The second thing I have to say is that there is illustrated in this result the single worst problem of neuropsychology or all psychological testing and that is the psychological tests or any test you give somebody samples their behavior only over a short period of time—usually minutes in your laboratory. The test of subjecting somebody to an attempt at a college education, however, takes four years. And you learn a lot about somebody when you give them that test that you can never learn about them when you give them the four-hour or the four-minute test—precisely because some disorders are disorders of temporal organization and of inability to plan ahead and sequence one's behavior over time. It will only be tests or procedures that sample over a long period of time that will ever disclose those I suspect. So there's an important caveat in those data.

SHAYWITZ: Let me say that I think that when people talk about attention disorders, they talk about dyslexia and dyslexia plus, I think that we, in my conceptualization (I'm not sure that other people would share this), we're really talking about two different conditions that often co-occur in the same child. You should all recognize that the term *attention disorder* is a relatively new one. It was coined in 1980 when DSM III was written; that's the *Diagnostic and Statistical Manual* that was published by the American Psychiatric Association. It was further confused and confounded in 1987 when DSM IIIR was published. The DSM IV, which is currently being written, will, hopefully, clarify some of the problems that we created in DSM IIIR. Primarily it will hopefully clarify the problem regarding attention disorder with and without hyperactivity.

But one should recognize that attention disorder, as it is currently used, is a diagnosis made purely on the basis of history—a history of children who have cardinal symptoms that relate to inattention, impulsivity, and hyperactivity. They may or may not have hyperactivity. Currently, that is the way attention disorder is defined. In contrast, most of us define reading disability on the basis of performance on reading tests.

So we are really almost talking about apples and oranges in a sense. We are making one diagnosis, ADD, on the basis of behavioral characteristics. We are making the other diagnosis, reading disability, on the basis of test scores. Again, I think when we talk about reading disability we are a lot more secure about the neuroanatomic foundations, work that many of these people on this platform have performed. We conceive of ADD and reading disability as two separate disorders that often co-occur. In epidemiologic studies, approximately 10% of children with attention disorder also have a learning disability. Those data are from a normal epidemiologic population. About a third of children with learning disability also have attention disorder. In referred populations, often 80% of cases have both disorders. So you need to know which population you are talking about. My take-home message suggests that you really ought to conceive of these problems as two separate problems that often co-occur in the same child.

DUANE: Then it is the purpose of your new Learning Disability Center to try to formalize and operationalize a definition of attention deficit disorders?

SHAYWITZ: Yes. The major question facing the field is, how do you define and differentiate these two disorders? Further confounding the issue is another problem diagnosis referred to as oppositional disorder. That leads to still more confusion!

LUBS: Unless there are other burning questions about this, I think there was one that was asked this morning that deserves to be addressed here and that's the question of response of particularly the children with familial dyslexia to the whole language approach and whether they also still need to learn the phonological approach. Here is another can of worms to discuss.

We did have a brief study of 20 children with familial dyslexia, about a quarter of them in our study. This was a one-on-one series of two to three sessions, three or four times a week for six weeks. It was a modified whole language approach. At least from the preliminary analysis of this investigation, they got strikingly better, mitigating two to three years worth of reading within that time. So whatever was done seemed to work very well. The problem is knowing what was done and why. How much of this was due to the one-on-one, the emotional support, the changes in self attitudes which were very striking when they occurred. The problem is (a) to make a study design to look at this and (b) almost certainly they do need more phonological skills. The difficulty is to do it in some different fashion from what we are now doing, perhaps taking into some recognition the things that I mentioned in terms of short-term memory and other ways in which different ways of approaching this speed of handling information or related factors. It needs to be done but we need to look at how to do it better. I'm guessing the answer is yes, we do not need to do both.

DUANE: Well you actually presage the conference or pre-conference meeting next year in Washington, DC for The Orton Dyslexia Society. At least it is under consideration that there might be a pre-conference symposium to look at this specific issue of educational intervention. Hopefully this will be done in a dispassionate way, investigating methodology and intervention in order to determine if there are hard data which would substantiate one or the other approach to any of a number of reading disorders.

WOOD: If I may take this opportunity to point out that we also, like Herb, are doing an intervention study, the results of which are being reported at this conference by my colleague, Dr. Felton.

DUANE: I believe that Dr. Liberman will also address the issue of phonological versus whole word approach at this conference.

I want to thank the Curtis Blake Center for their generous support so that this symposium could be held, as well as the members of the program committee who generated the notion of putting on this pre-conference symposium.

Summary

Drake D. Duane

One could rightly inquire, "If the purpose of this text, as the title suggests, is to discover the *reading* brain, why has so much been devoted to the brains of those for whom reading has been difficult?" There are two reasons. The first is that in science an understanding of the normal course of events often results from investigation of pathologic or exceptional conditions. The second is that reading disability is relatively common and can co-occur with high aptitude, with both perhaps being biologically engendered. Thus, the study of disability may simultaneously uncover the genesis of ability. The foregoing chapters present abundant data to support the hypothesis that both the morbid and the functional anatomy of a dyslexic person's nervous system differ from those for whom developing the skill to decode script is unhindered.

A curious fact is that most humans readily learn to speak but many never learn to read. Current estimates suggest that more than a third of our species are incapable of comprehending the written symbols of the language they speak. Less than five percent have developmental speech disorders. This discrepancy, in part, may have a biologic explanation. Early peripheral hearing deprivation or environmental deprivation of speech sounds lead to faulty oral language development. This type of auditory deprivation usually retards the acquisition of reading ability, as well. Early environmental exposure to speech sounds, and later to their written symbols, is required if reading skill is to develop.

Whether there is for reading a similar interaction between production and internalization, as the motor theory of speech perception suggests, is unclear (Liberman and Mattingly 1989). But most young readers reinforce what they have read by saying it out loud. For both speaking and reading, abilities previously acquired may be lost after puberty through localized injuries to the brain. For either speech or reading to be affected, the injury overwhelmingly affects the left hemisphere—predominantly anteriorly for speech, posteriorly for reading. Before puberty, acquired lesions must be much more widespread for either speech or reading to be hindered. It appears that the earlier the process that limits the development of speech occurs in brain development, the greater the probability there will be a similar interference with reading. This developmental association between speaking and reading may explain the prevalent concomitant anomalous oral language development in those with developmental reading disability.

In the absence of speech delays or cultural deprivation, what is the core discrepant dysfunction among the developmentally reading disabled? An obvious consideration is the role of vision and the visual system. Acquired adult disorders of reading commonly also impair the field of vision. In developmental disorders of reading, the association with vision is not clear-cut. There is no data to support a retardation in the acquisition of tactile perception for script among the congenitally blind. Children with developmental disorders interpreted as "visual perceptual," frequently encounter difficulties in learning to read." However, it is rare that reading problems occur in isolation in the visually perceptually handicapped. It has been suggested that the critical deficit might be an inability to integrate what is seen with what is heard at a symbolic level; that is, an inability to associate the mind's eye for graphemes and words with the mind's ear for phonemes and syllables.

The high frequency of no or low reading ability among humans, its relative difficulty in acquisition as compared with learning to speak, as well as the absence of written language in some primitive cultures raises the possibility of a natural selection for biologic attributes that may hinder reading acquisition on the one hand but perhaps promote survival on the other. These concerns validate an inquiry into reading *disability* in order to better comprehend the neurobiology of reading *ability*.

The work of DeFries, Lubs (both this volume), and others in the field of genetics underscores the fact that among the biological determinants of reading disability are heritable familial factors that by linkage analysis can now be associated with at least two distinct chromosomes, namely 6 and 15. These data pertain to those families in whom reading disorders involve at least three generations and meet criteria for a Mendelian dominant gene. It seems probable that these two chromosomal anomalies will be joined by others. A complex behavior such as reading would fit best with a polygenetic mechanism. What is not yet clear is whether this genetic pleuralism is associated with one or more than one anatomic or functional morphology. Is it possible that reading *giftedness* also may be genetically influenced? Or is it that the absence of chromosomal anomalies associated with reading disability allows reading to progress? The answer is unknown. Further, what biologic advantage these chromosomal deviations promote is yet to be discovered, but there may be some.

The introduction of twin studies in seeking answers to genetic questions raises questions about the twinning process itself. The true rate at which twinning occurs is unknown but may be as high as twenty percent. The much lower observed rate of twinning likely reflects the frequent occurrence of absorption of one of the twin pair. The late Norman Geschwind was intrigued with what appeared to be differential rates of twinning in various peoples and places. The determinants and significance of various rates of twinning are unknown. The opportunity to study large numbers of twins with reading disability affords the parallel opportunity to investigate other and perhaps related biologic features—for instance, the prevalence of one or more other biologically determined attributes such as rate of illness in reading-disabled versus other twin pairs. The study of twins reared apart convincingly shows how profound are the effects on behavior of shared genetic material (Bouchard et al. 1990).

Clarifying the role of gender in dyslexia is important and seems easy. Whether determined by sex chromosomes or sex steroids, this most profound biologic marker must not be neglected. It is confusing that the Yale investigation in the United States (Shaywitz et al. 1990) indicates equal occurrence of reading disability among males and females while the Isle of Wight study in England (Rutter et al. 1976) found a three and a half fold increase in males. Previous studies of impaired readers in the general classroom have shown an excess of boys over girls. This could reflect what Shaywitz and his colleagues suggest is an effect of the high co-occurrence of attention deficit hyperactivity disorder (ADHD) with reading disability. Their work suggests that ADHD is more prevalent in males than in females. An alternate possibility is that male selection bias reflects the reality that extremes in ability (giftedness or retardation) are more prevalent in males. If so, the observation still begs explanation. It is clear that there is a male referral bias to medical services for childhood developmental disorders. A recent personal survey of one hundred students referred to the Institute for Developmental and Behavioral Neurology for potential developmental disorders affecting academic performance revealed a four-to-one male-to-female ratio (Epcar and Duane in press). This gender bias was similar whether the diagnosis was ADHD alone, ADHD with reading disability, or reading disability in relative isolation. Thus, the occurrence of ADHD alone may not explain male referral bias. Aggressive behavior and social attitudes are other factors that may influence selection for medical referral. The former is also clearly more prevalent in males.

What is the role of gender in reading giftedness? It is suggested that a high level of reading ability in early grades is more prevalent in females. After grade school this gender distinction is less clear. A personal survey of one hundred male and one hundred female adults evaluated for non-developmental and non-behavioral neurological symptoms indicates 80% of the women, but only 30% of the men, recalled reading and spelling as their strongest academic aptitudes (Epcar and Duane in press). What factors mediate this type of gender effect, and are they social or biologic? These questions await clarification.

The gross anatomy of the brain in reading disability is consistent whether assessed by postmortem examination or magnetic resonance imaging (MRI) (Rumsey et al. 1986). A symmetric volume in the temporal regions is observed that correlates with equal width of the posterior hemispheres. This symmetric pattern is seen in less than 25% of the general population. Galaburda and his co-workers (this volume) have determined that this symmetry of the nervous system is a consequence of an abundance of neurons in the right hemisphere that survive the process of neuronal rejection usually completed by the age of four. Morphometric analysis of brain anatomy visualized by MRI is altered in congenital oral verbal agnosia, i.e., in children who have difficulty comprehending speech (Filipek et al. 1987). Interestingly, in this condition also, the alterations are bilateral and in the temporal region and consist of a symmetric reduction in cortical volume. What factors control these expansions or reductions in the volume of nerve cells of the brain's surface is not yet clear.

Whether by postmortem analysis or MRI, other gross morphologic changes, such as tumors or oddities of white matter hydration, are not commonly present and thus provide no further clue as to what miniscule or titanic event triggered the altered pattern of brain development. Assuredly its timing in ontogeny is prenatal. But is the brain for which reading is readily acquired necessarily asymmetric (as in the more common left-greater-than-right temporal plane surface area)? The answer is not known, but there have been reports suggesting that reading achievement can occur in individuals whose nervous system is symmetric or in which the symmetry pattern is reversed from the usual. What then are the critical characteristics which determine that deciphering script will be frustrating? Galaburda's work suggests that the answer lies at the microscopic level, and further that these microscopic changes may have induced the particular symmetric pattern observed in the dyslexic population.

The irregularities in the cortical mantle described by Galaburda and his co-workers (Galaburda, Rosen, and Sherman 1989) likely reflect multifocal fronto-Sylvian interruptions from the usual orderly migration of embryonic neurons. Among the speculations are that these migratory arrests result from humoral interaction ischemia secondary either to occlusion of the microvasculature on an autoimmune basis or the effects of fluctuations in maternal blood supply. However, there are several observations that complicate an interpretation. The first is that the microscopic pattern is not consistent between the two sexes. That is, the three female dyslexic nervous systems described by Galaburda either have no visible migratory cellular anomaly or a different pattern from that seen in the males. The fibromyelin plaques more probably relate to some form of circulatory interruption. Second is the observation by Adinolfi (in press) that it is improbable that maternal antibodies have any direct effect upon the developing fetus. Third is the work of Nowakowski (1988) which suggests that in mice the dysplastic cortex may be the direct product of genetic factors presumably operating in isolation. These ambiguities reinforce the necessity of further research both in animal models of cortical development and in human developmental mechanisms.

The issue of cerebral lateral asymmetry brings up the question of manual lateralization among those with reading disability. It is heuristic to consider the degree of hand preference and speed of limb movement as possible additional expressions of developmental patterns of brain anatomy. The belief that left-handedness for writing is more common among those with reading disabilities has not been proven. In dominantly inherited, twin or epidemiologic samples of dyslexic persons the rate of left-handedness is reportedly not increased above the general population (this volume). My own investigation suggests that rates of left-handedness among a variety of developmental disorders is not notably increased, but that weak right-handedness is unusually prevalent (Epcar and Duane in press). At all ages and in both males and females, Edinburgh laterality quotients below +75 occur in more than half of those with ADHD with or without reading disability and in those with isolated reading difficulty. Furthermore, partially inverted right-hand posture for writing is prevalent among those with developmental reading and spelling underachievement. A differential frequency of these physical markers among those with dominantly inherited dyslexia would suggest that there may be differences in brain organization in inherited versus non-inherited forms of reading disability. The question of sub-typing in reading disability could come to a classification based on differential cause.

As attempts are made to interpret functional anatomy by physiologic and metabolic techniques, it may be useful to determine manual lateralization, family history, and extent of developmental speech anomaly. These factors may contribute to the physiologic/metabolic variance. The technology of assessing functional anatomy is young and investigators in this area should be granted time to develop further investigative techniques that will influence the generation of specific hypotheses. A recent observation that is unlikely to change is that of the bilaterality of brain function in reading and other higher cognitive tasks. This bilaterality may explain why an early-in-life focal injury to the nervous system rarely, if ever, results in isolated reading impairment. If results prove congruous between different causes for dyslexia then the functional anatomy must represent the final common pathway for reading. Morbid and *in viva* gross anatomy represent the archeology of behavior; that is, they permit us to visualize the remnants of the ontogenesis of the nervous system—including its aging. Functional anatomy reflects the sociology of nervous system function as populations of neurons interact to produce community action. It may be functional anatomy that will best differentiate the reading from the non-reading brain.

Just as there may be manual preference, hand posture, brain anatomic, or brain physiologic concomitants in reading disability, there may be additional behavioral consequences to these biological events. Among these is the possible coexistence of disorders of attention or predispositions of the psyche that influence mood, levels of anxiety, and personality. As the Yale group has shown, ADHD is especially prevalent among boys with reading disability. Reading disability in isolation and ADHD in isolation are each associated with elevated rates of psychiatric diagnoses, particularly conduct disorder and depression (Brumback and Staton 1982; Rutter 1974). It is not clear if these turns of personality reflect the effects of school frustration, other environmental or familial factors, or are themselves the product of the biological states that create reading disability and/or ADHD (Duane 1989). Contrariwise, whether there are lower rates of these mental disorders among those with high reading achievement is not known. If rates of mental illness are lower, is it the experience of success or the biology of achievement or both that influences emotional outcome?

Since the major function of the brain is learning and adaptation, it seems plausible that limitations in adaptability have consequences for personality development. Successful intervention requires an understanding of what determines success in reading and success in living. Thus, understanding the biological constraints and differential features of the nervous system that learns to read readily, and the nervous system that does not, becomes essential. There already are lessons in medical intervention that have implications for future neurological interventions. Among these is the observation that while successful medicinal treatment for disorders of attention may promote more effective new learning and enhanced recall of verbal and/or visual information, changes in social behavioral patterns and the building of corpi of information require time. The need for time reflects the necessity of *relearning* behavioral patterns and filling gaps in collected information. New learning is more efficient than relearning. It follows that early learning is efficient learning. Accuracy in the early identification, whether biological or behavioral, of those at risk for reading disability offers the advantage of more efficient intervention and of minimizing secondary effects of reading failure.

The quest continues to identify the biological substrate that makes deciphering these pages difficult or easy. The joint presidential and congressional designation of the last decade of this millennium as "The Decade of the Brain" can bring that quest closer to a successful conclusion. Understanding the reading and non-reading brain may provide insights into other relationships of the human mind-brain.

REFERENCES

Adinolfi, M. In press. Maternal brain antibodies and neurological handicap. In *The Extraordinary Brain: Neurobiological Issues in Developmental Dyslexia,* eds. A. M. Galaburda, G. F. Rosen, and G. D. Sherman. New York: Plenum.

Bouchard, T. J. Jr., Lykken, D. T., McGue, M., Segal, N., and Tellegen, A. 1990. Sources of human psychological differences: The Minnesota study of twins reared apart. *Science* 250:223–28.

Brumback, R. A., and Staton, R. D. 1982. An hypothesis regarding the commonality of right hemisphere involvement in learning disability, attentional disorder and childhood major depressive disorder. *Perceptual Motor Skills* 55:1091–1097.

Duane, D. D. 1989. Neurobiologic correlates of learning disorders. *Journal of the American Academy of Child and Adolescent Psychiatry* 28:314–18.

Epcar, L., and Duane, D. D. In press. Pupillometry, sleepiness and vigilance in developmental disorders. *Neurology.*

Filipek, P. A., Kennedy, D. N., Caviness, V. S., Klein, S., and Rapin, I. 1987. *In vivo* magnetic resonance imaging-based volumetric brain analysis in subjects with verbal auditory agnosia. *Annals of Neurology* 22:410–11.

Galaburda, A. M., Rosen, G. F., and Sherman, G. D. 1989. The neural origin of developmental dyslexia: Implications for medicine, neurology and cognition. In *From Reading to Neurons,* ed. A. M. Galaburda. Cambridge, MA: MIT Press.

Liberman, A. M., and Mattingly, I. G. 1989. A specialization for speech perception. *Science* 243:489–94.

Liberman, I. Y., and Mann, V. 1981. Should reading instruction and remediation vary with the sex of the child? In *Sex Differences in Dyslexia,* eds. A. Ansara, N. Geschwind, A. Galaburda, M. Albert, and N. Gartrell. Towson, MD: The Orton Dyslexia Society.

Nowakowski, R. S. 1988. Development of the hippocampal formation in mutant mice. *Drug Development Research* 15:315–36.

Rumsey, J. M., Dorwart, R., Vermess, M., Denckla, M. B., Kruesi, M. J. P., and Rapoport, J. 1986. Magnetic resonance imaging of brain anatomy in severe developmental dyslexia. *Archives of Neurology* 43:1045–1046.

Rutter, M. 1974. Emotional disorder and educational underachievement. *Archives of Diseases in Childhood* 49:249–56.

Rutter, M., Tizard, J., Yule, W., Graham, P., and Whitmore, K. 1976. Research report: Isle of Wight studies, 1964–1974. *Psychological Medicine* 6:313–32.

Shaywitz, S. E., Shaywitz, B. A., Fletcher, J. M., and Escobar, M. D. 1990. Prevalence of reading disability in boys and girls. Results of the Connecticut Longitudinal Study. *JAMA* 264 (8):998–1002.

Index

(Page numbers in italics indicate material in tables or figures.)

AD. *See* Autosomal dominant (AD) dyslexia
ADD. *See* Attention deficit disorder (ADD)
ADHD. *See* Attention deficit hyperactivity disorder (ADHD)
Allergic disorders, 69–73
Angular gyrus
   activation in dyslexic subjects, 17–19, 20
   strategy differences between normal and dyslexic subjects and, 18
Animal models, 123–24, 128
Asthma, 71–72, 100
Atopic dermatitis, 100
Attention deficit disorder (ADD), 27, 45, 164–65, 175
   concurrent with learning disability, 176–77
   reading disability and, 6, 21
   without hyperactivity, 38
Attention deficit hyperactivity disorder (ADHD), 2–3, 5–6, 21
   conduct disorders and depression and, 184
   laterality quotients and, 183
   reading and, 5
Attentional disorders
   classification system for, 45–46, 47–48
   subtypes of, 49
Auditory Consonant Trigrams, 107
Autistic children, hypoplasia of cerebellar vermis in, 169
Autoimmune disorders, 69, 100
Autosomal dominant (AD) dyslexia, 89–93, 94–98, 113–16

immunological aspects, 98–102
magnetic resonance studies of, 108–111
neuropsychological aspects of, 105–107
positron-emission tomographic studies of, 111–13
vision and auditory studies of, 102–105

Blickman, J. G., 137, 138
Brain asymmetry, 14, 120–21, 182
   in dyslexic females, 102
   and symmetry in dyslexics, 122–27
   and symmetry and interhemispheric communication, 126
Brain donations, 165
Brain neurons
   asymmetry and number of, 123, 124–26
   excessive numbers of, 129
   migration of, 125, 126
   pruning of, 125, 126, 129
Brain(s)
   abnormally located cerebral cortex in, 152
   accuracy of spelling task in normal subjects and activation of left Wernicke's area of, 16–17
   border-defining contours of structures in, *146*
   "callosal" regions for morphometric analysis in, 152, *153*, 155
   cerebral asymmetry in, 110

Brain(s)—*continued*
  childhood and adult lesions of, 121
  corpus callosum, 109, 110, *111*, 142
  cytoarchitectural anomolies of, 14
  difficulty with elimination of developmental errors in, 129
  focal dysplasia in dyslexic, 127
  hemispheric shape variations of, 154–55
  injuries affecting speech and reading, 179–80
  language areas of, 120, 128, 129, 142
  language remediation and blood flow in, 172
  language task performance by reading-disabled subjects and posterior displacement of activation of angular gyrus, 17
  left temporal activation and reading task performance, 19–20
  meaning of cortical anomalies in, 127–28
  meaning of symmetry of, 122–27
  planum temporale asymmetry in, 120, 121, 122–23
  punctate activity in dyslexic, 167
  reading task-produced variations in regional metabolic activity of, 112
  regions involved in language functions, 120
  shape of, 143–44, 148, *149*
  specialization of cerebral hemispheres of, 141
  structural anomalies of developmental origin, 133
  symmetry of planum temporale in dyslexic, 108
  volume changes in, 143, 148–54
  See also Brain asymmetry; Cerebral blood flow; Computed tomography (CT); Left hemisphere; Magnetic resonance imaging (MRI) *entries*
Broca, Paul, 120

Caviness, V. S., 142
Cerebral blood flow
  influence of language tasks on

  patterns of, 15–17, 112
  with word-hearing and reading tasks, 156
  See also Regional cerebral blood flow (rCBF)
Childhood dyslexia
  adult functional neuroimaging phenotype of, 13–20
  adult neuropsychological phenotypes of, 10–13
Chromosomal markers, 83, 92, *98, 99, 100*
Chromosomal trail loci, 82–83
Chromosomes, genetic linkage and behavior in meiosis, 91
Chromosome 6, 74, 75, 77–79, *82*, 115–16, 180
  evidence for linkage between reading disability and, 83
  familial dyslexia and, 72
Chromosomes 13 and 14, possible dyslexic genes on, 97
Chromosome 15, 74, 115–16, 180
  linkage between specific reading disability and heteromorphisms on, 192, 193
  locus for dyslexia on, 92
  multipoint analyses of linkage between specific reading disability and markers on, 77, *78*, 79
  two-way analysis with reading disability and heteromorphism on, 75–77
Classification systems, research and, 32–33
Cognitive deficits, reading related, 10–13
Cognitive functions and abilities
  number of neurons and, 129
  reading and writing and, 105–107
  sex and, 172
Colorado Reading Project, 53–54
  twin/family study of, 54–62, 68–72, 83–84
Computed tomography (CT), 134, *135*, 139–41
  quantitative analyses of (in dyslexia), 141–42
  radiation exposure with, 140
Confrontation naming, 5

Cross concordance analyses, 69–73
CT. *See* Computed tomography

Decoding of words, reading deficit
    attributed to, 4
DeFries, J. C., 56, 57–59, 60, 61
Developmental disorders in child-
    hood, 133
CT and MRI and, 139–41
Down syndrome, 174
Dyslexia
    basis for larger number of males
        with, 96
    classification of, 32–33
    definition of, 93
    evolution of concept of, 28–29
    focus on underlying process as ap-
        proach to defining, 13,
        20–21
    gender and, 7–8, 9, 171, 181
    importance of family history of,
        115
    lack of functional test for, 113–14 ✓
    lack of operational definition of, 1
    language and, 29–31
    maternally-passed, 171
    probable most frequent form of in-
        heritance of, 89
    race and, 8–9
    sex differences in, 115
    sex-linked (absence of), 162
    study of autosomal dominant,
        89–93, 113–16
    See also Autosomal dominant dys-
        lexia; Childhood dyslexia;
        Chromosome 6; Chromo-
        somes 13 and 14; Chromo-
        some 15; Family studies;
        Reading disability
Dyslexic individuals
    anomalous organization of left
        hemisphere in, 13–14
    temporal lobe tumors in, 175
    temporal visual information pro-
        cessing deficit in, 105
    visual sensitivity in, 104
Dystonics, handedness in, 161

Environmental influences, 66, 67, 68
    on correlation between ortho-
        graphic coding and word
        recognition, 67, 83

Epilepsy in students with learning
    problems, 166–67

Family studies, 53, 54–62, 69–70,
    74–83
    See also Autosomal dominant dys-
        lexia; Sib pair method; Twin
        entries
FAS test, 105, 109
Female fetuses, spontaneous abor-
    tion of, 171
Filipek, P. A., 137, 138, 142
Fletcher, J. M., 33
Francis, D. J., 33
Fulker, D. W., 57, 59

Galaburda, A. M., 99, 102, 142
Gender ratios
    at birth, 171
    and impaired reading ability, 163,
        169–70
    in special dyslexic groups, 163–64
Genes
    linkage analysis to localize, 73
    nature of linage of, 91
Genetic correlation between pho-
    nological coding and word
    recognition, 68, 83
    using categorical measures, 69
Genetic covariance, 65
Genetics, frequence of recombina-
    tions in, 91
    See also Chromosome *entries*; Fam-
        ily studies; Linkage anal-
        ysis; Twin pairs
Geschwind, N., 99, 102, 121
Gillis, J. J., 61

Handedness, non-right-, 99
Helper cells, 101
Heritable influences in correlation
    between phonological cod-
    ing and word recognition,
    68, 83
    See also Linkage analysis
Hyperactivity, ADD without, 38

Immune diseases in females, 171
Immunological differences, epi-
    demiology of, 68–73

Kennedy, D. N., 142

Laterality, 161
Learning, major influences on, 48, 49
Learning disabilities (LD), 27, 45
    classification system for, 42–44, 45, 47–48
    handedness and, 161
Left hemisphere
    normal asymmetry of posterior temporal planum of, 14
    spelling task accuracy and blood flow to Wernicke's area in, 16–17
    See also Brain(s)
Levitsky, W., 121
Liberman, I. Y., 30
Linkage analysis, 73–74
    aim of, 114–15
    See also Genes; Genetic entries
LOD (Log of the Odds of Linkage), 74, 91

Magnetic resonance-based blood flow/blood volume studies of the brain, 156–57
Magnetic resonance imaging morphometry
    applications of, 148–54
    computerized method of, 144–48
    rationale of, 142–44
    sources of error in, 154
Magnetic resonance imaging (MRI), 108–111, 134
    clinical diagnosis vs. research application of, 141
    clinical use in developmental disorders, 138–41
    in diagnosis of developmental learning or language disorders, 157
    principles of, 135, 136, 137–38
    quantitative analyses of (in dyslexia), 141–42
    spatial resolution of, 142
    three-dimensional brain reconstructions using, 168
Menick Syntactic Comprehension Test, 105–106, 107, 108
Migraines, 70, 168–69
Morris, R. D., 33
MRI. See Magnetic Resonance Imaging (MRI)

Multiple regression analysis of twin data, 56–62, 65, 83

National Institute of Child Health and Human Development (NICHD), 53, 54
Neurolinguistic tests, correlations between reading measures and, 37–38
Neuronal migration, 125, 126
    forming upper cortical layers of brain, 14
Neuropsychological test battery, 106

Ojemann, G. A., 14
Olsen, R. K., 64, 65, 66
Oppositional/conduct disorders, 177
    classification system for, 45–46
Orthographic coding, genetic and environmental factors in, 66
Orthographic tasks. See Spelling tasks
Orton, Samuel T., 29

Phonemic awareness, 5
Phonological coding, 63–65
    genetic covariance between word recognition deficits and, 68
    heritable deficits in, 66
Phonological tasks, 63–65
Positron-emission tomography (PET), 111–13, 167, 173
    to observe brain processes during single word activation, 156
Psychological tests, significance of length of, 176

Race, reading scores and, 8–9
Rapid naming, 5
Reading ability
    gender ratios and impaired, 103
    language-based theory of, 30
Reading ability in childhood, cognitive skills in adulthood and, 10–13
Reading disability behavioral and genetic analysis and, 65–66
    best evidence for heritable nature of, 59
    brain and, 182
    chromosome 6 and, 74, 75, 77–79, 82, 83

chromosome 15 and, 75–77, *78, 79*
cognitive correlates of, 6–7
evidence for genetic etiology of, 56, 57–58, 59, 60–61, 83
immune disorders and, 69–73
impaired decoding of words and, 4
IQ and, 11
issues concerning cognitive and biological mechanisms in, 31–32
possible genetic subtype associated with atopic disorders, 83
referral bias in, 170
related to confrontation naming, phonemic awareness, and rapid naming, 5
research on subtypes of, 68–69
significance of definition of, 170
specific, 75
study of first-grade, 3–9
subtypes of, 49
test for genetic etiology of, 56, 57–58, 60–61
two-way analysis with chromosome 15 heteromorphisms and, 75–77
See also Dyslexia
Reading-disabled individuals, absence of normal left-greater-than-right asymmetry in posterior temporal planum, 14
See also Dyslexic individuals
Reading-disabled and no-reading disability groups, patterns of differences between, 38–39, *40, 41, 42*
Reading and language skills and processes in reading-disabled and normal groups, 62–65
Reading measures, correlations between neurolinguistic tests and, 37–38
Reading skill, early exposure to speech and, 179
Referral bias, 170, 181
Regional cerebral blood flow (rCBF) Novo Cerebrograph 32C system

for, 15–16 133-Xenon method of monitoring, 15
See also Cerebral blood flow
Research, classification systems and, 32–33

School performance, neurobehavioral disorders and, 28
Sex ratios. *See* Gender ratios
Sib-pair method, 81–82
Skinner, H. A., 33
Smith, S. D., 90, 91, 97
Specific reading disability (SRD), 75
linkage map of chromosome 6 with, *82*
See also Dyslexia; Reading Disability
Spelling task, 63–64
focal activation of left Wernicke's area and accuracy of, 16–17, 19
See also Orthographic coding
Spoken language, inability to understand, 151
Suppressor cells, 101

T-cells, 101
Twin data, multiple regression analysis of, 56–62, 65, 83
Twin pairs, 69, 71–73
comparison of concordance rates of reading disability in (as test for genetic etiology), 56
determining zygosity of, 55

Vellutino, F. R., 30
Verbal auditory agnosia (VAA), 151–53
Verbal fluency, dyslexics with good, 107
Vision, pattern detection and motion detection and, 103–104
Visual sensitivity, specific difference between dyslexic and normal readers in, 104

Wadsworth, S. J., 61
Whitaker, H. A., 14
Whole language approach, children with familial dyslexia and, 177

Word deafness, VAA and adult pure, 151

Word recognition, 63
  differential heritability of deficts in, 66–68
  environmental factors in, 67, 83
  genetic covariance between phonological coding and deficits in, 68, 83
  genetic influence on, 66